End of Life in Care Homes

Please r

End of Life in Care Homes: A Palliative Approach

Edited by

Jeanne Samson Katz

Sheila Peace

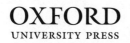

OXFORD
UNIVERSITY PRESS

Great Clarendon Street, Oxford OX2 6DP

Oxford University Press is a department of the University of Oxford.
It furthers the University's objective of excellence in research, scholarship,
and education by publishing worldwide in

Oxford New York

Auckland Bangkok Buenos Aires Cape Town Chennai
Dar es Salaam Delhi Hong Kong Istanbul Karachi Kolkata
Kuala Lumpur Madrid Melbourne Mexico City Mumbai Nairobi
São Paulo Shanghai Taipei Tokyo Toronto

Oxford is a registered trademark of Oxford University Press
in the UK and in certain other countries

Published in the United States
by Oxford University Press Inc., New York

A catalogue record for this title is available from the British Library

Library of Congress Cataloging in Publication Data
(Data available)
ISBN 0 19 851071 3

10 9 8 7 6 5 4 3 2 1

Typeset by Newgen Imaging Systems (P) Ltd., Chennai, India
Printed in Great Britain
on acid-free paper by
T.J. International Ltd., Padstow

Preface

This book explores the possibilities for improving the care of older people dying in residential and nursing homes. It comes at a time when there is much public debate in the United Kingdom about which statutory authorities should have the responsibility of providing and funding chronic and end-of-life care for older people in all settings. Whilst much of the data presented here was collected in the United Kingdom, similar issues face provision of care to residential settings in other Western countries (e.g. Clare and De Bellis 1997).

The development of palliative care during the last third of the twentieth century revolutionized the experiences of dying people themselves and their carers in modern societies (see Oxford Textbook of Palliative Medicine). The palliative care movement has created an environment where dying, like childbirth, has slowly come full circle insofar as those concerned have had choices about, for example, sites of care or types of treatment restored to them. However even at the turn of the century real choices about end-of-life care are available primarily to certain categories of dying people—those who are young or middle-aged, educated, articulate, and for the most part probably middle-class.

This book examines a category of disadvantaged dying: those people disenfranchised by physical and sometimes mental deterioration. These older people live in institutional settings, often with little opportunity to exercise choice about such mundane, yet central activities such as when to take a shower, or schedule meals; additionally they rarely have access to the services offered by palliative care.

Whether palliative care services should be accessible to people dying from diseases other than cancer is a contested issue. In addition there is debate as to whether it is appropriate to deliver palliative care to the nursing and residential sector. An argument against delivering palliative care to people dying from conditions other than malignancies is that 'palliative care' as we now know it, could be diluted. This book will present some of these debates; however the central tenet is that there are aspects of palliative care that, given the right circumstances, are transferable to people living with chronic disabling conditions or dying in institutional settings; indeed these aspects of palliative care may indeed be generalisable to most environments, to different groups of dying people including those who are physically or mentally disabled.

Having established some broad guidelines for adapting certain aspects of palliative care to these settings, the book will suggest some strategies for health workers. This is not a textbook in palliative medicine nor even in palliative care—both these fields are more than adequately catered for by a number of publications, the most comprehensive of which is the Oxford Textbook of Palliative Medicine. What this book sets out to do is to identify possibilities for delivering palliative care to the older sector of the population who despite suffering from a multiplicity of chronic conditions currently receive rather patchy terminal care, particularly in nursing and residential homes.

A central principle of palliative care is the multidisciplinary team and the encouragement of positive interchange of ideas amongst different groups of professionals as well as with informal carers. Therefore this book is aimed at palliative care practitioners, primary health care teams and home staff who are most likely to have contact with dying people in residential settings.

Drawing on research data (Sidell *et al.* 1997; Katz *et al.* 1999, 2000; Komaromy *et al.* 2000) the book will describe common scenarios of dying in nursing and residential homes. Care staff face challenges in dealing with practical, health and emotional issues as well as managing the rest of their work. These include addressing care needs of dying older people, surviving residents, relatives and colleagues. Carers work within considerable constraints and often have little training especially in end-of-life care. Through the use of extensive case studies and shorter vignettes examples of more effective working will be identified. We will also explore issues of access for these settings to palliative care services in the United Kingdom as well as in the United States.

This book can be read from start to finish; but it also can be a resource in particular topics. For this reason some concepts and findings from research data are repeated.

Acknowledgements are due to a number of people and organisations. First and foremost to those older people and their carers who have participated in several of the studies reported in this book and to the Department of Health who funded them. Second, to the authors who generously agreed to contribute to this book. Third, to our colleagues at the School of Health and Social Welfare At The Open University where much debate takes place about addressing the needs of disenfranchised populations. Fourth, to Pauline Byrne and Serena Stewardson who with wonderful good humour and commitment to this project have assembled this manuscript extremely carefully. Penultimately, to Catherine Barnes and others at Oxford University Press who saw the need for a book on this topic and cheerfully prodded us for some time to produce a book proposal! And finally to our spouses, our children, and definitely not forgetting our parents for providing us with sustained support, stimulation, encouragement and welcome distractions.

Jeanne Samson Katz and Sheila Peace
The Open University

References

Clare, J. and De Bellis, J. (1997) Palliative care in South Australian nursing homes. *Australian Journal of Advanced Nursing*, **14**(4), 21–8.

Katz, J.T., Komaromy, C., and Sidell, M. (1999) Understanding palliative care in residential and nursing homes. *International Journal of Palliative Nursing*, **5**(2), 58–64.

Katz, J.T., Komaromy, C., and Sidell, M. (2000) *Investigating the Training Needs in Palliative Care*. Unpublished report for the Department of Health.

Komaromy. C., Sidell, M., and Katz, J.T. (2000) The quality of terminal care in residential and nursing homes. *International Journal of Palliative Nursing*, **6**(4), 192–204.

Sidell, M., Katz, J.T., and Komaromy, C. (1997) *Death and Dying in Residential and Nursing Homes for Older People: Examining the Case for Palliative Care*. Report for the Department of Health.

To our parents, Renée and Ernest Samson
and Johanna and Reginald Peace

Contents

List of contributors

Stephen R. Connor
Vice President, Research, Development
and Finance
The National Hospice and Palliative
Care Organization
1700 Diagonal Road
Suite 625
Alexandria, VA 22314, USA

David Field
Visiting Professor
Department of Epidemiology and
Public Health
University of Leicester
22–28 Princess Road West
Leicester LE1 6TP

Katherine Froggatt
Head of Macmillan Practice
Development Unit
Macmillan Practice Development Unit
School of Nursing and Midwifery
University of Southampton
Highfield
Southampton SO17 1BJ

Jeanne Katz
Senior Lecturer
School of Health & Social Welfare
The Open University
Walton Hall
Milton Keynes MK7 6AA

Carol Komaromy
Lecturer in Health Studies
School of Health & Social Welfare

The Open University
Walton Hall
Milton Keynes MK7 6AA

Miriam S. Moss
Senior Research Scientist
Polisher Research Institute
Abramson Center for Jewish Life
Philadelphia Geriatric Center
261 Old York Road, Suite 427
PO Box 728
Jenkintown, PA 19046, USA

Sidney Z. Moss
Project Director
Polisher Research Institute
Abramson Center for Jewish Life
Philadelphia Geriatric Center
261 Old York Road, Suite 427
PO Box 728
Jenkintown, PA 19046, USA

Sheila Peace
Senior Lecturer
School of Health & Social Welfare
The Open University
Walton Hall
Milton Keynes MK7 6AA

Moyra Sidell
Senior Lecturer
School of Health & Social Welfare
The Open University
Walton Hall
Milton Keynes MK7 6AA

Chapter 1

Introduction

Jeanne Katz and Sheila Peace

The end of life takes place in different situations and settings. At the beginning of the twenty-first century we have an ageing population with changes in family and household composition that influence how and where older people may be cared for. In the United Kingdom, health and social care policies have resulted in a decline of long stay hospital beds and a greater focus on rehabilitation, intermediate care and independent living which have altered the balance between people living in their own homes and those living in residential care homes and nursing homes. These long-term care facilities have become places where many older people find themselves as they approach death. Similar patterns are found in the United States where health trends, such as the ageing population, and pressures to reduce the costs incurred in hospital admissions and home care, indicate that nursing homes are likely to become the location where people die. Indeed in the United States, the probability that death would occur in a nursing home increased from 18.7 per cent in 1986 to 20 per cent in 1993 (Zerzan *et al.* 2000).

The types of and funding for residential accommodation for older people vary within the countries of the United Kingdom (Christie 2002) and differ too from facilities in the United States, Australia (Zinn 2002), and other western nations. Residential care and nursing home settings do not, by type, offer uniform services to different categories of dying people. As will be elaborated in the next chapter, the philosophy of many of these settings does not necessarily incorporate preparing residents for death or training carers in terminal care or even how to handle chronic conditions.

At some levels the dearth of information about what happens to older people, deteriorating and dying in all settings, is surprising given the publicity which has accompanied the development of the hospice and palliative care movements in English-speaking societies. Not only is there little research into the ways in which older people die (and indeed causes of death), but also there is little debate in relation to the appropriate policies which might determine the types, possible sites and quality of care of dying older people. Specifically, there has been little discussion about how the enormous strides made in pain control might contribute to the care of older people in nursing and residential settings. In parallel there has till recently been relatively little debate about the advantages or disadvantages of applying, adopting or adapting specific principles of palliative care to people of all ages dying of non-malignant disease in all settings.

The case for using palliative care for people dying of diseases other than cancer is the focus of a comprehensive volume on this topic (see Addington-Hall and Higginson 2001). Similar to the groundbreaking discussions in that work, this is one of the first books to focus exclusively on the possibilities of applying appropriate aspects of palliative care to caring for older people dying in residential and nursing home settings. Like Addington-Hall and Higginson (2001), we as authors have only in relatively recent years become concerned with end-of-life issues for older people in residential care, despite having become interested in palliative care through doctoral studies focussing on strategies used by health professionals caring for people dying of cancer (Katz 1996) and many years of research into the residential sector catering for older people (Peace *et al.* 1982, 1997; Willcocks *et al.* 1986).

This book and the various research projects reported herein have emerged from assumptions (and now some evidence) that first, by the end of the twentieth century the care of older people dying in institutional settings was not of the same standard as those dying in other settings, and second, that palliative care may have something concrete to offer. As this book focuses on how we could bring about improvement in the care of dying older people through considering which aspects of palliative care would be most useful, it is important to consider how and why palliative care has developed and what it purports to be.

What is palliative care?

Many medical, nursing and social science texts describe the nature and philosophy of palliative care. However most of these texts start from the premise that palliative care is primarily applicable to the care of people dying from what is perceived to be terminal illness. This usually refers to malignant conditions, although palliative care has gradually become accepted as appropriate for looking after sufferers of amyotrophic lateral sclerosis, more commonly known in the United Kingdom as motor neurone disease. The one uniform thread running through many of these texts is that the dying individual is incurable and *likely to die within a loosely predicted time frame*. Another assumption is that palliative care is best delivered in a hospice or the dying person's own home, and in some cases in hospitals.

With such large numbers of people dying in residential, nursing and long-term care facilities, why is it that palliative care has not reached this potentially huge audience? In order to understand how this anomaly has arisen it is important to briefly rehearse the history of the modern hospice and palliative care movement. The beginning is often associated with the work of Dame Cecily Saunders in the United Kingdom, who when working as a nurse noted the distress in which many people died in public hospitals in the United Kingdom. In order to address some of these difficulties she retrained as a social worker and then qualified as a physician before specializing in pain control. Her project, to establish a home for dying people, materialized in 1967 when St Christopher's Hospice was opened in Sydenham, outside London. The focus of her concern and that of her followers was initially to address the intense pain and isolation that people dying of cancer suffered in the terminal phase of the illness. Her work could be seen as part of a crusade to ensure that as many aspects of a dying person's suffering as possible were alleviated and she coined the phrase 'total pain'. Total pain encapsulated many of her goals, to ensure that not only were the physical needs of dying people addressed but also that their social, emotional, psychological, practical, and spiritual needs were also met.

Cancer was an obvious candidate for palliative care. Particularly in the 1960s and 1970s most cancers were seen to be incurable and sufferers were reported to experience intractable pain. In contrast to the most frequent causes of death (cardiovascular disease including stroke) it was relatively possible to predict the disease trajectory of someone with cancer. Additionally a sizeable, though minority proportion of people with cancer are young or middle aged, and therefore accompanied by the concept that these deaths are not timely. Publicity was easy to obtain particularly where cancer patients were people with 'high social value', young mothers, talented young adults, all with much to live for, and potentially leaving behind bereft children and families.

The emotional attraction to cancer causes was helped by many research studies in the middle of the twentieth century which revealed that particularly in state-run institutions (e.g. National Health Service Hospitals in the United Kingdom, public hospitals in the United States) people dying of cancer were experiencing extremely painful deaths (Glaser and Strauss 1965, 1968; McIntosh 1977). Health professionals were reportedly unable to address their physical pain, and to a large extent removed themselves from emotional involvement with dying people (ibid.; Sudnow 1969). Many explanations have been offered for this phenomenon, some connected with the 'curative' focus of medical training and socialization, others associated with the then poor knowledge of pain relief.

Through publicizing the fate of those dying of cancer, honing her own pain control skills, and embarking on an extraordinarily successful crusade against the medical establishment, yet with the support of the health service and some conventional medical practitioners, Cecily Saunders founded the Hospice movement with St Christopher's. She saw this as a place where research, teaching, and in-patient care could collaborate and it became the mecca for the international hospice movement which developed apace. Services and facilities for dying people in addition to conventional in-patient care were developed in tandem. These included day care, and most importantly, domiciliary care. Indeed many hospice services in the United Kingdom started as domiciliary services before building purpose-built facilities. In the United States most services started as, and have remained as domiciliary services.

As services evolved so did titles and names. Once the international movement took on, it became apparent that in French the word 'hospice' had a pejorative connotation, so the Canadians, who too were pioneers in this area, suggested the term palliative, rather than hospice. However, the Americans had already adopted this term, so it sticks there and is used primarily in the United Kingdom to describe the in-patient building.

There are different types of hospice and palliative care services in the United Kingdom all of which are delivered free of charge to the user; these services are funded by the National Health Service (NHS) primarily as well as by charitable contributions. The first type is the 'hospice building', a purpose-built or adapted building housing in-patient beds. These may be voluntary or independent hospices (registered charities), (some of which may be partly funded by the NHS); the NHS palliative care units or centres; Macmillan Cancer Care units funded by the charity, Macmillan Cancer Relief; and Marie Curie Centres and Sue Ryder homes funded by the charities of the same names. Patients are usually admitted to an in-patient unit for one of three reasons, in order to achieve symptom control, to give dying people or their informal carers respite (a few days relief with assured quality of care) or for terminal care when dying people have reached the end stage. Hospices provide a range of services for dying people in addition to conventional in-patient services—for example, day care services, beauty therapy, complementary therapies, and bereavement care.

The second type is *palliative care in domestic settings*. The conventional home care and more extended home nursing service known as 'hospice at home' may be provided by multidisciplinary teams containing palliative medicine consultants, nurses, social workers, and other professionals allied to medicine or by individual or groups of palliative care clinical nurse specialists

(CNS) known generically as Macmillan nurses (even where they are not funded by Macmillan Cancer Relief). 'Hospice at home' may be provided to avoid admission to an in-patient unit or for respite care or crisis management (Hospice Information 2002). Forty per cent of the domiciliary palliative care nursing services in the United Kingdom are provided out of voluntary hospices, the remainder is provided by Community NHS trusts (including Macmillan nurses). Also Marie Curie Cancer Care has over 4000 part-time nurses providing 24 h one-on-one care for people with cancer in their own homes.

Third, there are *Hospital Palliative Care Teams*, sometimes known as Support or Symptom Control Teams who provide symptom control, pain relief and emotional support to inpatients and outpatients as well as support and advice to medical, nursing and paramedical colleagues as well as informal carers such as relatives and friends. These teams may include all or any of the following—doctors, social workers, nurses, and clergy. Many of these services are provided by a single Macmillan nurse.

In 1980, there were 62 hospice services in the United Kingdom including home care teams; by 2002 there were 208 adult in-patient units providing 3029 beds, 243 day-care services, 78 'hospice at home' services, 100 hospital support nurses and 221 hospital support teams providing home care (Hospice Information Directory 2002). Expanding from initially providing services for adults with cancer only, 4.8 per cent of the patients have non-cancer diagnoses, including HIV/AIDS, motor neurone disease, heart disease, and stroke (Hospice Information website 2002). There are also home care and in-patient facilities for children. During the 1990s there were both dedicated and general hospice units caring for people with HIV/AIDS but many units closed due to advances in HIV medication.

So what package of palliative care do these hospice and palliative care services offer? The following box contains the widely cited WHO definition of palliative care as well as the definition and statements from the Canadian Palliative Care Association which encapsulate palliative care as we envisage it for older people in residential settings.

The aims of most palliative care organizations can be summarized as follows:

1 To provide symptom control and pain relief for the dying person, avoiding inappropriate treatment.

2 To create a support system for dying people, providing social, emotional, spiritual and practical care in an individualized way enabling them to exert control, independence and choice, an opportunity to live as actively as

Palliative care

+ Affirms life and regards dying as a normal process
+ Neither hastens nor postpones death
+ Provides relief from pain and other symptoms
+ Integrates the psychological and spiritual aspects of patient care
+ Offers a support system to help patients live as actively as possible until death
+ Offers a support system to help the family cope during the patient's illness and in their own bereavement (WHO 1990).

Hospice palliative care

It aims to relieve suffering and improve the quality of living and dying. Hospice Palliative Care is appropriate for any patient and/or family living with, or at risk of developing a life-threatening illness:

+ Due to any diagnosis
+ With any prognosis
+ Regardless of age
+ At any time they have unmet expectations and/or needs, and are prepared to accept care (Canadian Palliative Care Association Website, last updated Oct. 2001).*

* This website is now called Canadian Hospice Palliative Care Association: www.chpca.net.

possible, and participate in decisions relating to managing problems. This might include negotiating the most appropriate place to die (home, hospice or hospital).

3 To provide emotional, spiritual and practical care for the dying person's family and friends during the illness, and after death (bereavement care).

4 To establish a team, with good communication between the members, including the dying person and his or her family.

5 To provide support and expert advice to those caring for dying people (hospital team, GP, social worker, psychologist, district nurse, clergy, dietician, volunteer, chiropodist or physiotherapist) irrespective of the site of care, whether home, hospital, residential home or hospice (Katz and Komaromy 2000).

6 To undertake research and provide education for those caring for dying people.

Palliative care only works when all the carers subscribe to a common goal as articulated in the *Introduction to Palliative Care in the Home*:

> The goal of palliative care is to achieve the best quality of life for patients with incurable life-threatening diseases. Palliative care provides relief from pain and other distressing symptoms and offers a support system to help the family cope during the patient's illness and bereavement. Terminal care is that part of palliative care which takes place in the last days of life, when the aim is to enable the patient to die with dignity.

(Doyle and Jeffrey 2000: 1)

The wider society sees palliative medicine as providing a combination of pain relief and a secure, controlled environment for those at the terminal stage of illness.

Palliative care is not a monolithic concept, and over the past ten years has redefined itself into specialist palliative care and the palliative approach. Specialist palliative care is usually practised by professionals with training and specific qualifications in palliative care or considerable experience through extensive work with dying people and their families. Specialists in palliative care can come from several disciplines, including, for example, physicians from a number of medical specialities, nurses from a variety of backgrounds and social workers. They work alongside conventional health providers in most settings where dying people are cared for. This includes, as indicated above, working in hospices; in people's own homes with community nurses and primary care teams; in nursing homes working with nursing home staff; and in general, specialist, and community hospitals working in conjunction with radiotherapists, oncologists, surgeons and physicians.

The palliative approach on the other hand is practised by generalists and takes the principles of palliative care as articulated in the WHO definition and the aims cited above and applies them to the care of any sick person regardless of the nature of their illness. The debates about the relevance of this approach to caring for people dying of non-malignant conditions are discussed in Addington-Hall and Higginson (2001), and these turn on many issues, including training and resource allocation. We intend to extend these debates to the particular section of the community on which this book focuses. In particular we hope to consider how cultures of care emanating from traditions grounded in maintenance and more currently 'rehabilitation' could potentially refocus to incorporate particular aspects of palliative care to ensure better medical, social and nursing care of older people dying in nursing and residential homes. We are not criticizing the different culture of care in residential environments which already care for dying older people, but are suggesting that through education and training, care staff, relatives and managers could benefit from the now extensive experience of caring for dying people in other settings.

The Open University studies

Research studies have been undertaken in the United States, Australia, and to a lesser extent in the United Kingdom on the way in which dying people are cared for in *nursing homes* (Keay and Schonwetter 1998; Frogatt 2000, 2001*a,b*; Maddocks and Parker 2001). Because of the paucity of research studies about people dying in *residential care*, particularly in the United Kingdom this book draws extensively on data derived from two Department of Health funded studies based in England and undertaken by three of the contributors working at The Open University, Jeanne Katz, Carol Komaromy, and Moyra Sidell. The first study, referred to in the book as OU Study (1) took place between 1995 and 1997 (Sidell *et al.* 1997; Katz *et al.* 1999, 2000*b*; Komaromy *et al.* 2000; Sidell *et al.* 2000; Katz *et al.* 2001). This study aimed to:

(1) ascertain if the principles and practices of palliative care had permeated the ethos of residential and nursing homes for older people;

(2) assess the feasibility of applying appropriate aspects of palliative care to the care of people dying in these settings.

It used a multi-method approach to data collection using both quantitative and qualitative methods.

OU Study (1)—methodology (1995–7)

The *first stage* of the study was a postal survey sent to a randomized sample of 1000 residential, nursing and dual-registered homes (not including homes for elderly, mentally infirm people (EMI)) in the Northwest, Southeast, and West Midlands of England in 1996. 412 usable questionnaires were returned. Data collected included demographic information about residents; frequency of transfers out of the homes, provision of staff training in terminal care, and also home managers' concepts of palliative care. The *second stage* comprised of interviews conducted on site with 100 home managers randomly sampled from the 412 responses to the postal survey. Interviews were taperecorded and included structured and semi-structured elements covering a range of topics including staffing arrangements and training issues. Through exploring the management of death and dying of the last three residents to die in the home, home managers explained their philosophy of care for dying residents. They focused on defining the resident as dying, the terminal care provided and the relationships with staff external to the home, other home staff and relatives of the dying residents. They also reflected on the appropriateness of palliative care

OU Study (1)—methodology (1995–7) *(continued)*

for people dying in residential care. A purposive sample of 12 homes was selected as the sample for the *third stage*. These reflected a spread of size, type and geographical locations and also a range of philosophies and practices. Participant observation, informal and tape recorded interviews were used to ascertain how death and dying is managed and to elicit, where possible, the views of all participants. Information about caring for dying residents was collected from over 400 people in the case studies including residents, relatives, home staff of all ranks (those providing hands-on care were usually called 'carers' or 'care assistants'), 22 general practitioners, 12 community nurses, and eight specialist palliative care nurses.

(Sidell *et al.* 1997)

The same research team also undertook what is referred to in this book as OU Study (2) (Katz *et al.* 2000a). This two-year study (1997–9) followed the first and investigated the training needs of the disciplines involved in providing care to older people dying in residential and nursing home settings. The main aims were to ascertain staffs' needs for training, explore methods of meeting them, and subsequently to devise a set of training materials to address them. Once again data were collected using both quantitative and qualitative methods.

OU Study (2)—methodology (1997–9)

Stage one involved setting up and running 15 focus groups of internal and external professionals caring for residents in residential, nursing and dual registered homes. Twelve of those homes were selected from those used in the first research study but not case study homes (Sidell *et al.* 1997). The purpose of the focus groups was to:

- conduct an audit of previous training, skills and resources available to staff
- ascertain the different perspectives and skills each type of carer brought to this work
- determine the type of training that carers require
- explore understandings of palliative care with carers.

The skills and background questionnaire data from group members and field notes from the group discussions were analysed in relation to training needs. This analysis identified five different topic areas suitable for developmental

OU Study (2)—methodology (1997–9) *(continued)*

training workshops. These included: an introduction to palliative care; pain control, and ethics; communication; cultural, religious and spiritual needs, and bereavement care and support. *Stage two* entailed developing multimedia training materials in six topic areas: a foundation in palliative care; communication; pain control; ethics, culture, and bereavement. The *third stage* involved the running of *30 workshops in 17 homes* in all the topic areas to test the materials. The purpose of the workshops was to evaluate the appropriateness of the materials to the needs of the participants in terms of:

- content—including level and relevance
- context—of the home as a training setting and the composition of the training group
- process of the learning experience including: the activities and facilitation; the impact of the workshops on the participants' knowledge and skills in palliative care.

Further self-administered questionnaires were given to those participating in the workshops. These included an evaluation to test out the appropriateness and effectiveness of the training materials and the ways in which they were delivered. In *stage four* the training materials were evaluated according to:

- the appropriateness of the materials for the needs of the participants
- the appropriateness of the content of these materials for the different types of settings
- how the materials developed could be used—for example, whether they could be used by lone individuals or only in groups, and whether or not a facilitator was required
- an assessment of the process of the training workshops and whether the academic level of the materials had been appropriate for the participants
- a measurement of whether participants thought following workshops that aspects of palliative care were indeed appropriate for their work settings.

The *final stage* of the development process was the production of a set of draft training materials (Katz *et al.* 2000*a*). Subsequent further modification of these materials was funded by the Department of Health and Macmillan Cancer Relief will be publishing them in 2003. The details of these materials are discussed in Chapter 8.

The structure of this book

In this book we build up a picture of dying in residential settings for older people in the United Kingdom. We examine the reasons for the limited access to palliative care services for older people with conditions other than cancer (Addington-Hall and Higginson 2001) specifically in relation to those dying in residential settings (Zerzan *et al.* 2000). Now that 'grey power' is a force to be reckoned with, might this situation change and could books like this help carers to act effectively as advocates of those older people unable to represent themselves? The following chapters should provide useful information about the needs of older people dying in these settings, and raise the important issues for policy and practice.

In Chapter 2, Peace chronicles the history of residential and nursing home provision for older people and contextualizes this in relation to the development of health and social service policy in the United Kingdom. Sidell and Komaromy look at the nature of the population which dies in these settings and examine the reasons why staff are not always able to provide adequate care for dying residents. The central concept of the 'dying trajectory' is raised in this chapter. Using data which emerged from the OU Studies, Katz, in Chapters 4 and 5, describes the challenges of caring for dying residents, the constraints faced by staff and implications for managing a home and on staff morale of a death. Komaromy explores in Chapter 6 how carers construct their interactions with relatives and other residents following a death in the home. The roles played by external health workers, particularly general practitioners, community nurses, and specialist palliative care teams in caring for dying residents are explored by Katz in Chapter 7.

Sidell in Chapter 8, through describing the development of training materials in palliative care for home staff, delineates the conditions essential for their effective delivery. Through the use of two detailed case studies, specific aspects of the principles and practices of palliative care which lend themselves for adaptation to care homes are demonstrated by Katz in Chapter 9. Moving across the Atlantic, Moss, Moss, and Connor in Chapter 10 explore the needs of those people residing in the nursing home sector in the United States and the roles, which hospice has begun to play in caring for dying residents. In Chapter 11, Field and Froggatt examine some of the debates in relation to providing palliative care services for older people not necessarily dying of cancer and residing in care and nursing homes. They look at alternative ways of delivering palliative care to these settings which recognize and value their own unique and different culture and begin the process of summing up the arguments raised in this book. In conclusion, Peace and Katz suggest that relationships and resources are the key concepts to be considered in relation to addressing the palliative care needs of older people dying in care settings.

References

Addington-Hall, J.M. and Higginson, I.J. (eds) (2001) *Palliative Care for Non-Cancer Patients*. Oxford University Press, Oxford.

Canadian Palliative Care Association (2001) (www.cpca.net).

Christie, B. (2002) UK divided as Scotland and introduces free personal care for older people. *British Medical Journal*, **324**, 1542.

Doyle, D. and Jeffrey, D. (2000) *Palliative Care in the Home*. Oxford University Press, Oxford.

Froggatt, K.A. (2000) *Palliative Care Education in Nursing Homes*. Macmillan Cancer Relief, London.

Froggatt, K.A. (2001*a*) Palliative care in nursing homes: Where next? *Palliative Medicine*, **15**, 42–8.

Froggatt, K.A. (2001*b*) Life and death in English nursing homes: Sequestration or transition? *Ageing and Society*, **21**, 319–32.

Glaser, B.G. and Strauss, A.L. (1965) *Awareness of Dying*, Aldine Publishing Company, Chicago.

Glaser, B.G. and Strauss, A.L. (1968) *Time for Dying*, Aldine Publishing Company, Chicago.

Hospice Information (2002) *Minimum Data Sets—National Survey 1999–2000 document* (www.hospiceinformation.info).

Katz, J. (1996) Nurses' perceptions of stress when working with dying patients on a cancer ward, in G. Howarth and P.C. Jupp (eds) *Contemporary Issues in the Sociology of Death, Dying and Disposal*. Macmillan, London, 124–36.

Katz, J.T., Komaromy, C., and Sidell, M. (1999) Understanding palliative care in residential and nursing homes. *International Journal of Palliative Nursing*, **5**(2), 58–64.

Katz, J. and Komaromy C. (2000) *Workbook 2: Caring for Dying People*. The Open University, Milton Keynes.

Katz, J.T., Sidell, M., and Komaromy, C. (2000*a*) *Investigating the Training Needs in Palliative Care*. Unpublished Report for the Department of Health.

Katz, J.T., Komaromy, C., and Sidell, M. (2000*b*) Death in homes: Bereavement needs of residents, relatives and staff. *International Journal of Palliative Nursing*, **6**(6), 274–79.

Katz, J., Sidell, M., and Komaromy, C. (2001) Dying in long term care facilities: Support needs of other residents, relatives and staff. *American Journal of Hospice and Palliative Care*, **18**(5), 321–6.

Keay, T.J. and Schonwetter, R.S. (1998) Hospice care in the nursing home. *American Family Physician*, **57**, 491–4.

Komaromy, C., Sidell, M., and Katz, J.T. (2000) The quality of terminal care in residential and nursing homes. *International Journal of Palliative Nursing*, **6**(4), 192–204.

McIntosh, J. (1977) *Communication and Awareness in a Cancer Ward*. Croom Helm, London.

Maddocks, I. and Parker, D. (2001) Palliative care in nursing homes, in J. Addington-Hall and I. Higginson (eds) *Palliative Care for Non-Cancer Patients*. Oxford University Press, Oxford, 147–57.

Peace, S.M., Kellaher, L.A., and Willcocks, D. (1982) *A Balanced Life: A Consumer Study of Life in 100 Local Authority Old Peoples' Homes*. Research Report 13. CESSA, Polytechnic of North London, London.

Peace, S.M., Kellaher, L., and Willcocks, D. (1997) *Re-evaluating Residential Care.* Open University Press, Buckingham.

Sidell, M., Katz, J. T., and Komaromy, C. (1997) *Dying in Nursing and Residential Nursing Homes for Older People: Examining the Case for Palliative Care.* Report for the Department of Health. Open University, Milton Keynes.

Sidell, M., Katz, J.S., and Komaromy, C. (2000) The case for palliative care in residential and nursing homes, in D. Dickenson, M. Johnson, and J.S. Katz (eds) *Death, Dying and Bereavement.* Sage 2nd edition, London, 107–21.

Sudnow, D. (1969) *Passing On: The Social Organization of Dying.* Prentice-Hall, Englewood Cliffs, NJ.

Willcocks, D.M., Peace, S.M., and Kellaher, L. (1986) *Private Lives in Public Places.* Routledge, London.

World Health Organization Expert Committee (1990) Pain Relief and Palliative Care, *World Health Organisation Technical Report Series,* 804. WHO, Geneva.

Zerzan, J., Stearnes, S., and Hanson, L. (2000) Access to palliative care and hospice in nursing homes. *JAMA,* **284**(19), 2489–94.

Zinn, C. (2002) Australia: Government subsidizes long term care by up to £22,000 a year. *British Medical Journal,* **324**, 1543.

Chapter 2

The development of residential and nursing home care in the United Kingdom

Sheila Peace

Introduction

Reflections on the past history of institutions tell us a great deal about how their present day culture has evolved. In this chapter, the scene is set for understanding the position of present day nursing homes and residential care homes as places where older people live and die; a position formed of people and places where practice has evolved within a specific history. Attention here will focus on the last two centuries until the present day. This has been one of two stories—for nursing homes, and for residential care homes—coming together at times and being treated separately at others. It has not been until the recent Care Standards Act 2000 that we have seen both terms being replaced by the words 'Care Homes' for institutions which provide accommodation, together with nursing or personal care (Standard 3 CSA 2000) and the development of National Minimum Standards (DoH 2001a). The reality of this unity is yet to be seen.

In this chapter, I begin by considering the historical development of both services before focussing on the past 25 years. During the latter period recognition of the changing nature of our ageing society has developed alongside ideological debate and policy development concerning the provision of long-term care for older people. Consideration will be given to the current characteristics of this provision within residential care homes and nursing homes examining the nature of the people and the places that make up these services, and recent changes in policy that have affected them. Finally, the chapter will end by reflecting on how the culture of care has evolved within these settings and how issues regarding dying and death have only relatively recently been recognized as key aspects of the purpose of long-term care (Abel-Smith 1964: 1).

Early developments

But first to return to the past, whilst groupings of poor and destitute people have been recorded over the centuries (Townsend 1962), it is common to acknowledge that the English Poor Laws imposed the first legal responsibility on society for the care of the aged. During the eighteenth and nineteenth centuries parallel histories of voluntary hospitals and workhouses evolved. Abel-Smith (1964) reports that when hospitals were first categorized in the 1851 census only 7619 patients were enumerated. Until that time illness of any kind was usually managed at home where people, especially the sick poor, were cared for by kin. People with financial resources could seek care within voluntary hospitals set up by founding charities, the majority of which were in London (Abel-Smith 1964: 46).

From the times of the 1834 Poor Law, a system based on 'lesser eligibility' meant that those without employment, money or shelter, and those who were sick and without family support, were obliged to seek 'relief'. 'Indoor' relief was given through workhouses where men and women were separated and where people laboured for their keep. Consequently, during the nineteenth century there were a greater number of sick people living in workhouses than the gradually developing hospitals. Under the Poor Law Amendment Act of 1851, Boards of Guardians who oversaw the workhouses at parish level were empowered to subscribe to voluntary hospitals and send pauper patients to them. However few did and hospitals became more concerned with cases of acute rather than chronic illness. In 1861, 11 000 patients were enumerated in voluntary hospitals whilst 50 000 sick persons were under the care of the workhouse medical officer (Abel-Smith 1964: 34).

Older people would live in the workhouse until they died:

> ... If the old man was dying they'd maybe let the old lady come and see him or vice versa. And at the end they used to have a jingle:
>
> > Rattle his bones over the stones;
> > He's only a pauper that nobody owns.
>
> And that's what it was. That's why they built the cemetery up close to the work-house, so they could take them over on a barrow.
>
> (Albert Funnel, a child in Brighton in the 1900s
> quoted in Thompson *et al.* 1990: 38)

Outside of the workhouse system many people had to pay for their burial. In the nineteenth century, those managing developing hospital institutions did not want to incur the expense of funerals and people often had to guarantee funeral expenses before admission (Abel-Smith 1964: 11–12).

The late nineteenth century saw the beginning of the reform of the work-house system and a gradual acknowledgement that it was the duty of the state to provide hospitals for the poor—pauper hospitals which later became public hospitals. As Abel-Smith states, 'the principle of need had triumphed over the principle of less-eligibility' (1964: 96).

Moving out of the Victorian era, the early twentieth century saw the gradual emergence of a liberal and socialist philosophy developing the labour movement and recognizing the importance of family life, and the needs of children, the unemployed, and the sick. However, the institutional arrangements of older people were slow to change (Townsend 1962). The report of the Royal Commission on the Poor Laws, in 1909, indicated that almost half of the institutional population living in workhouse accommodation were older residents (Peace *et al.* 1997: 7). At this time recognition of the needs of an ageing society had not surfaced as a twentieth-century issue, older people in these situations were part of the sick poor who may or may not be in need of health care. Their situation within the workhouse system was due to their poverty and not their age.

However, the debate concerning 'to pay' or 'not to pay' for health care continued. Small pox epidemics led a wider variety of people with different financial status to seek hospital care which led to the development of convalescent care (Abel-Smith 1964). From the 1880s onwards separate nursing homes, pay hospitals and pay beds developed:

> The movement to find accommodation for paying patients had arisen largely out of the nursing reform movement: it became more advantageous to provide institutional care for those of modest income who could not be conveniently nursed at home. This led to the creation of separate nursing homes and Home Hospitals.
>
> (Abel-Smith 1964: 150)

Nursing homes offered a range of medical assistance—maternity care and surgical treatment which included the needs of some older people. These became procedures that could no longer be carried out in a person's own home. Abel-Smith reports that: 'In 1891 there were about 9500 beds in England and Wales in nursing homes and convalescent homes; by 1911 this number had increased to 13 000' (1964: 189) which then doubled to 26 000 by 1921 (1964: 339). The quality and provision within nursing homes was hotly debated throughout the early twentieth century. But it was not until the 1920s that the conditions of some of these homes and the care provided especially for the chronic sick which was causing concern to nurses and medical officers of health paved the way for the appointment of a Select Committee on Nursing Homes (Registration) (Abel-Smith 1964: 338–42). Evidence to the Committee (Ministry of Health (MoH) 1926) reported on the terrible circumstances of some patients:

> They frequently develop bed sores due to prolonged neglect. They are rarely washed. The bed linen is changed at very infrequent intervals, even when soiled.

> The rooms are verminous. No adequate protection is taken to prevent dissemina-
> tion of contagious or infectious diseases.
>
> (Abel-Smith 1964: 341)

As a consequence the Nursing Homes Registration Act 1927 introduced the first system of registration and inspection for these privately run homes (see discussion of regulation, p. 30).

The historical development of the workhouse and the nursing home provides important background for the ideology concerning the development of the National Health Service and issues of payment for health care. When commenting on the views of the Select Committee of Nursing Homes, Abel-Smith points to the class-based divisions between those living in nursing homes and workhouses—stating:

> The real problem was the 'senile and chronic sick' among the class of persons
> who did not desire to incur the stigma of a Poor Law institution. For this group
> the committee recommended 'the provision of proper paying accommodation by
> the local authorities'.
>
> (Abel-Smith 1964: 342)

But to return to the workhouse population. It was not until the late 1920s that a reclassification of workhouse institutions saw the creation of Public Assistance Institutions (PAIs) and the transference of powers from the Poor Law Board of Governors to county and borough councils. In 1939 there were still nearly 400 public assistance institutions, accommodating 149 000 residents, 60 000 of whom were classified as sick—a majority of whom were older people (MoH 1939).

Circumstances during the period of the Second World War brought change. Various factors came together: there was a need to discharge patients from existing hospitals in order to accommodate war casualties which meant that many frail and sick elderly people were forced either to seek admission to a PAI or to fend for themselves; some older people living in cities became homeless due to air raids, and the consequence was the overcrowding of PAIs. Different forms of small hostel accommodation were suggested at this time (Means and Smith 1983) and the findings of the 1947 Nuffield Survey Committee of PAIs recommended a radical move away from mass establishments to small homes with 25–30 places (Nuffield Survey Committee 1947). Consequently, Section 21 of the National Assistance Act 1948, placed a duty on local authorities to provide 'residential accommodation for persons who, by reason of age, infirmity or any other circumstances are in need of care and attention not otherwise available to them'; and the annual report of the MoH in 1948–9 recorded the demise of the workhouse with these words:

> The old master and inmate relationship is being replaced by one nearly approaching that of hotel manager and his guests.
>
> (MoH 1950: 311)

In framing this Act, a distinction was made between nursing homes and residential care homes that focused on accommodation or 'board and lodging' in relation to residential homes.

The postwar years

In the postwar years building materials were in short supply and many public sector residential homes for older people were developed out of upgraded workhouses and old, converted buildings. The small home of up to 35 places was an ideal at this time. In 1948 PAIs were still providing indoor relief for 130 000 people in England and Wales. These were split into three groups: 100 PAIs were transferred to the MoH for use as hospitals under the National Health Service Act; a further 100 went to local authorities to be used as residential homes, and the remaining 200 were called 'joint user establishments' as they housed a mix of sick people and others and were therefore divided between Regional Hospital Boards and local authorities (MoH 1949; Townsend 1962).

Concern over the well-being of individuals was only beginning to emerge and little regard was being given to those who cared for them. Whilst the National Assistance Act 1948 had not sought to exclude ambulant older people from publicly supported residential care homes, gradual shifts in policy saw provision targeted at those who were more frail. Guidance issued during the 1960s and 1970s drew distinctions between health care and social care—seeing residential care homes as primarily for those people failing to cope at home even with domiciliary care and yet not in need of 'continuous care by nursing staff' (see Judge 1986: 7). The official concerns during this time had not been related to the objectives of care but rather to the development of new homes; the number of people to be accommodated, and subsequent costs. Indeed, concerns over costs and the number of users led to economies of scale and a proposal for 60-bedded homes (MoH 1955).

Whilst local authorities became the major providers of residential care homes, a small but growing number of older people lived in nursing homes and residential homes run by owners/proprietors in the private and voluntary sectors registered with local authorities (see regulation, p. 30). In the postwar period these were the relatively small homes commonly utilizing large domestic houses extended for this purpose.

Table 2.1 Number of residential institutions, beds, residents, and residents of pensionable age—England and Wales, 1 January 1960

Type of Institution or Homes	Institutions or Homes		Beds		Residents of all ages		Residents of pensionable age	
	Number	%	Number	%	Number	%	Number	%
Former public assistance	309	9.3	36 934	33.3	34 781	33.3	29 615	31.0
Other local authority	1105	33.1	36 699	33.3	35 139	33.7	33 677	35.2
Voluntary	815	24.5	25 491	23.0	24 360	23.3	22 410	23.5
Private	1106	33.2	11 643	10.5	10 120	9.7	9825	10.3
Total	3335	100	110 767	100	104 400	100	95 527	100

Note: Some local authorities were unable to supply detailed information about residents (and residents of pensionable age) in voluntary and private homes and the numbers were assumed to be in the same ratio to total beds as in other areas.

Source: Townsend, P. (1962) *The Last Refuge*. Routledge and Kegan Paul, London. Table 6, p. 43.

Learning from Townsend

In 1960, Peter Townsend carried out his seminal study of residential care homes and institutions—*The Last Refuge* (1962). At this time he shows that in England and Wales there were 3335 residential institutions or homes accommodating 110 767 people—95 527 (86 per cent) being over pensionable age. A third of the residents were accommodated in former public assistance institutions (31.0 per cent); a third in local authority homes (35.2 per cent) and the final third split between voluntary (not for profit) (23.5 per cent) and private (for profit) provision (10.3 per cent) (see Table 2.1). He was not concerned with nursing homes.

Whilst, *The Last Refuge* forms a key text for understanding why the quality of life experienced by older people living in this form of accommodation and care needed to be reformed, it also gives us a limited understanding of what happened to older people at the end of their lives. In discussing his survey data, Townsend comments on the flowing admission and discharge of residents. Taking the period of one year, 1959, his analysis of data from 147 local authorities shows that 35 803 people were admitted to homes from their own homes, hospitals, and other residential institutions whilst 33 785 people were discharged (Townsend 1962: 51). Of the later group 25 per cent died within the homes whilst 37 per cent were discharged to hospitals and 38 per cent to other settings. He comments that the death rate varied widely from 3 per cent of residents to 26 per cent in different homes with the explanation being seen in varied hospitalization rates, and reports that this was at odds with the government policy of the time which advised 'local authorities to avoid hospitalisation if possible during terminal illness' (Townsend 1962: 52). He also noted that the Ministry of Health's definition of the responsibilities of the welfare authority includes the care of those elderly persons:

> who have to take to bed and are not expected to live more than a few weeks (or exceptionally months) and who would, if in their own homes, stay there because they cannot benefit from treatment or nursing care that can be given at home, and whose removal to hospital away from their familiar surroundings and attendants would be felt to be inhumane.
>
> MoH Circular 14/57 [Footnote (1) 1962: 52]

In his more detailed study of specific accommodation, Townsend visited a wide range of institutions—old workhouses (39), local authority postwar homes (53), private homes (42), and voluntary homes (39). Interviews were undertaken with all officers-in-charge and residents across the homes and details were collected on all the social and physical characteristics of residents and issues to do with staffing, amenities and furnishings. Within his analysis he has something to say about how dying and death was handled in these various institutions.

Within the old workhouses he found a few who commemorated the death of individual residents whilst in the main there was little acknowledgement:

> Generally, however, a death was hushed up and the body removed swiftly and silently. No doubt the staff were anxious to avoid giving cause for anguish but they failed to realize that by their attitude they provoked insecurity. Many of the old people were aware that their lives were drawing to a close. Some were fearful, it is true, but most were reconciled to the idea or even welcomed it. The death of others disturbed them less than the concealment of it. And the way death was treated was perhaps a crucial test of the quality of the relationship between staff and residents. Dishonesty in this most serious of matters created distrust over minor affairs. And to avoid the rituals observed in an ordinary community had other consequences. Prompt removal of the body was not only, old people felt, the final indignity which a resident suffered but it gave no chance to those who were left of paying their last respects to someone who had lived amongst them, however remotely, and of thereby giving a little more strength, dignity and feeling to the slender relationships between those who continued to share the life of a ward. Perhaps these observations have less force when considering some hospital environments. But for old people in residential institutions they seem to be of considerable importance.
>
> (1962: 96)

In postwar local authority homes he comments on the way in which a room may be separated and used either for committee meetings or as a 'sick bay' or 'death room'. For one matron this room was used for people who were dying, 'I put them in the front lounge if they are dying. I don't let them die in a room *with others'.* (1962: 115). He describes a range of scenarios from many homes where death is hidden, nothing is said and no one goes to the funeral, to a few homes where residents are informed, may visit the body and say goodbye, club together for a wreath, and go to the funeral if they wish to. The psychological and social consequences of death were little understood and Townsend felt that the quality of death in homes symbolized failure. He says:

> There's a hush for an afternoon but no one talks about it and everything's the same by the evening. 'They take it in their stride. Old people don't seem to care.' We came to believe that this reported reaction symbolized the fundamental failure of the post-war Homes. They did not create a substitute community or a network of social relationships which could sustain a sense of individual purpose or pride.
> (Townsend 1962: 148)

The last twenty-five years

But the failure to recognize the needs of those experiencing life and death continued. In 1975, there were 195 100 residential places (66 per cent local authority; 13 per cent private; 21 per cent voluntary) and 24 000 nursing home places run by the private and voluntary sectors. In addition there were 49 000 long stay geriatric places in hospitals (Table 2.2).

This was the situation of the long-term care sector for older people at the start of a period of immense ideological change in policy development since the break-up of the workhouse system. It also came at a time when demographic and household change within an ageing society was now beginning to be recognized.

The ageing society

From the beginning of the last century the population of the United Kingdom has been increasing, life expectancy has improved considerably with a longer life for women over men, and as a consequence so has the number of people over 65 years of age (Social Trends 2002). The number of older people has doubled since 1931 and whilst there will be some minor rises and falls, this trajectory of growth will continue until 2030 when it will slow down (The Royal Commission on Long Term Care (RCLTC) 1999: 13–14; DoH 2001). During the first-half of the twenty-first century the greatest relative increase in older people will be amongst those over 85 years and it is the experiences of these people that will have the most important implications for long-term care given that more than 20 per cent of this age group live in residential care and nursing homes (Laing 2002).

Factors that will affect how frail older people live their lives are varied and relate to personal health, social support, financial position, and service development through political action and ideological influence (see Fig. 2.1).

- *Individual:* growing number of very old people, especially women; the compression of morbidity may lead to a shorter period of chronic illness and disability prior to death (see Royal Commission on Long Term Care, p. 15; Sidell 1995).
- *Social support:* changes have occurred in the pattern of family structures and responsibilities of work and at home; several million people provide hours of unpaid care especially children/children-in-law and spouses; some families live at a distance from each other.
- *Economic position:* the improved financial position of many older people means that some are making a positive choice over long-term care; housing circumstances throughout life can affect decisions over accommodation and care in later life.
- *Ideological influence:* the1980s saw an increasing popular support for a pluralist approach to welfare; in the 1990s and moving into the twenty-first century growing reliance on the market within health and social services.
- *Political action:* early stimulation of independent sector provision through public funding; an attack on institutional care through community care legislation; changes in funding; increased regulation and standard setting.
- *Service development:* increased pressure on long-stay hospital beds; more effective use of acute hospital beds; development of intermediate care and rehabilitation services; increased direction through National Service Framework for Older People.

Fig. 2.1 Factors which have affected the demand for long-term care in later life— 1980 onwards.

Source: Derived from Peace et al. Re-evaluating Residential Care. Open University Press. 1997; Long Term Care Commission 1999; Sidell 1995; Laing 2002; DoH 2001.

Providing accommodation, and social and health care

The election of the Thatcher Conservative government in 1979 formed a dividing line in the history of residential care for older people. Until the 1980s local authority old people's homes formed the main avenue for those moving into residential care. But in the 1980s, residential care homes started becoming market commodities. Of particular importance were the 1980 Supplementary Benefits (Requirements) Regulations which enabled people entering private residential care to obtain financial support through board and lodgings payments, thus enabling many poorer old people who qualified for income support to enter more easily using public funds. This system was channelled through the benefits system, without requirement for people's care needs to be assessed by the Local Authority.

These financial changes were fundamental to the exponential increase in private sector provision. As Table 2.2 shows, between 1983 and 1985, the number of private residential places grew by 60 per cent; and yet between 1985 and 1990 public provision of residential care fell by 8.4 per cent whilst places in voluntary homes remained relatively static and private provision increased dramatically by 82 per cent. Overall, during the 1980s, provision overtook demand as predicted by demographic change (see Fig 2.1) (Higgs and Victor 1993; Laing 2002).

Table 2.2 Nursing, residential, and long stay hospital care of elderly, chronically ill, and physically disabled people, places by sector, UK 1970–2001

	Residential places			Nursing home places		Long stay geriatric places
	LA	Private	Voluntary	Private	Voluntary	
1 April						
1970	108 700	23 700	40 100	20 300		52 000
1975	128 300	25 800	41 000	24 000		49 000
1980	134 500	37 400	42 600	26 900		46 100
1983	136 500	54 700	45 300	29 000		46 900
1985	137 100	85 300	45 100	38 000		46 300
1987	135 500	114 600	42 200	52 000	8300	43 000
1990	125 600	155 600	40 000	112 600	10 500	47 200
1995	79 700	169 300	56 700	193 400	17 900	33 000
1998	68 000	180 700	53 500	203 200	18 200	24 500
2000	60 000	185 000	54 500	186 800	18 000	21 000
Proj. 2001	57 400	185 100	55 100	178 800	18 000	19 700

Note: The private or 'for-profit' and the voluntary or 'not-for-profit' sectors became known as the independent sector.

Source: Adapted from—Laing (2002) Healthcare Market Review 2001–2, Laing and Busson, London, p. 173.

Growth continued to a peak of 321 200 residential places in 1990 which was followed by lower percentage growth in the residential sector. These changes followed the implementation of the 1993 NHS and Community Care Act reforms which sought to reduce the 'perverse incentive' towards institutional care through the facilitation of home care (CM 849 1989). In 1993 state funding for care homes was transferred to local authority budgets and care management was developed to assess individual needs for both home care and institutional placements. Of course this assessment did not include those people who paid for their own placement in these settings—known as 'self-funders'.

In contrast to the residential sector, the nursing home sector saw a gradual increase throughout the 1980s and 1990s with a particularly marked growth since 1985–6, especially within the private sector. In 1985, the ratio of residential care home places to nursing home places stood at 7 to 1; but by 1990 this had become 3 to 1 and projected figures for 2001 put this at 1.5 residential care home places to 1 nursing home place. The changing fortunes of the nursing homes sector reflect the steady decline in NHS geriatric and psychogeriatric beds, particularly since 1989 and the increasing nursing needs of residents. Consequently, whilst beginning from a much lower historic base than residential care homes, this sector has increased dramatically from 123 000 beds in 1990 to a high of 224 400 (+82 per cent) in 1997 followed by a more recent decline to 196 800. The residential care home sector has seen a more long-term gradual decline of approximately 7 per cent of places from 1990 to 2001 with projected beds of 297 700 (all figures based on Laing 2002).

These more recent changes relate predominantly to the characteristics of the institutional population and developments within the long-term care industry. In particular, residential care homes and nursing homes have been affected by:

(1) the debate and consequential funding arrangements concerning accommodation and personal and health care—which followed the Royal Commission in 1998 (RCLTC 1999). Free nursing care was introduced in England and Wales from October 2001; whereas free personal and nursing care has been adopted in Scotland;

(2) the development of intermediate care and rehabilitation services[1] to enable some older people to move from hospital or their domestic home into a residential care or nursing facility for a short stay in order to re-establish/maintain a level of supported independence within the community (Laing 2002);

(3) the introduction of national regulatory bodies working with National Minimum Standards for provision.

All of these initiatives have impacted on the financial requirements of accommodation and care that are beginning to change the long-term care market.

The characteristics of people and places

But what do we know of the characteristics of older people and staff living and working within care homes today?

The residents

The literature concerning institutional care for older people shows us that certain people are more likely to become residents than others. Factors affecting

---

[1] The National Beds Inquiry in 2000 reported that two-thirds of hospital beds were occupied by people aged 65 years and over and that a proportion of older people occupying acute hospital beds could have been treated in alternative facilities. These findings led to the development of intermediate care and rehabilitation services (Laing 2002).

the likelihood of current placement include advancing age, gender, and being of white British culture (Bebbington *et al.* 1996; Bauer 1996), social factors such as living alone, levels of care needed, social support, and housing (Sinclair 1988; Sinclair *et al.* 1988), and health issues relating to a decline in physical and cognitive functioning and the ability to undertake activities of daily living (Levin *et al.* 1994; Brown *et al.* 1997). It is the combination of these factors which lead some older people to no longer cope, or wish to cope, with living in their own homes. Currently they are most likely to be of white ethnicity (Bauer 1996) although the ageing of minority ethnic groups and their experience of changing social support will alter this situation.

Of all those aged 65 years and over, approximately 4 per cent live in care homes. However, this percentage increases dramatically with age, so that over 20 per cent of people over 85 years live in care homes with at least three quarters of residents being women (Laing 2002). More than half of the residents living in independent sector care homes currently have their fees paid by local authorities whereas 30 per cent are self-funders (Netten *et al.* 2001; Laing 2002). A crucial factor in the future development of these communal services is the level of resources made available from central government to local authorities to fund community care and enable people to stay at home if that is their choice (Laing 2002).

But, as we have seen, the circumstances of people in later life are changing and this will affect where people live and die. Data from the 2000 Health Survey for England adds to this picture (Bajekal 2002). In Bajekal's study, 2400 people living in care homes were interviewed as well as 1600 people living in private households. This study showed that two-thirds of permanent residents had moved from private households whereas 14 per cent moved from hospital, and that the majority had been living in the care home for between 2 and 4 years. Many of the people admitted to care homes were older women who had been living alone. Whilst residents were less likely to have social support than people living in their own home, 64 per cent were visited by their relatives or friends at least once a week.

The health status of older residents is particularly revealing when compared with people living in their own homes. Whilst self-assessed general health did not differ greatly, residents were more likely to be underweight, suffering from anaemia and a majority suffered from long standing illness and severe disabilities. The survey reports that three in four of all residents in care homes were severely disabled although, as expected, severe disability rates were lower in residential care homes (c. 70 per cent) than dual-registered homes (85 per cent) and nursing homes (91 per cent). Whilst, difficulty with walking and using stairs was the most common condition reported for both men and women, senile dementia was the most frequently reported cause of disability in care homes. Ninety-five per cent of people living in private households showed no signs of cognitive impairment whereas 49 per cent of those tested in care homes did, of which a third showed signs of having severe impairment. This was especially true of residents aged 80 years and over.

Consideration of the health and social circumstances of many residents in care homes show that whilst they are a diverse group, they do reveal a range of vulnerabilities which undermine their personal resources. It is therefore not surprising that mortality statistics for 1999 show that among those people over 85 years of age whilst the greatest number die in hospital, a comparable number of older women die in other settings including nursing homes and residential care homes (see Table 2.3). The future development of assessment for older people will have an important part to play in how choices are made over where people end their lives as outlined in the National Service Framework for Older People (DoH 2001*b*; 2002).

Staffing

It was not until the 1980s that legislation determined that a registered medical practitioner, or first level registered nurse should be in charge of a nursing home (see regulation, p. 30) and for many years there has been little information about the exact staffing levels of residential care homes and nursing homes which relate to the levels of resident need for personal and nursing care. The recent move to further develop pre-placement assessment and determine nursing and personal care will impact on staffing (DoH 2002).

The National Minimum Standards for Care Homes (DoH 2001*a*) say this:

> It is necessary to achieve a balance between drawing up standards which are specific enough to avoid the need for local negotiations, but which are broad enough to apply to the diverse nature of the clientele catered for (e.g. those who are physically frail; those who have dementia). Drawing up standards for staffing exemplifies some of the greatest difficulties of this kind. Where residents have a high level of dependency (in relation to capacity to perform the activities of daily living), staffing levels will need to reflect the needs of those residents. Where they require significant nursing attention, the skill mix of the staffing establishment must be adjusted accordingly. Residents with dementia also require care from appropriately skilled staff—and so on. In determining appropriate staffing establishments in all care homes, and in nursing care homes in particular, the regulatory requirement that staffing levels and skills mix are adequate to meet the assessed and recorded needs of the residents at all times in the particular home in question must be met.
>
> (DoH 2001*a*: 33)

These comments reflect current debates about multidisciplinary assessment (DoH 2002); discussions which reflect the need for a quality workforce where training is expected. Again the National Minimum Standards for Care Homes for Older People state that '*Staffing numbers and skill mix of qualified/unqualified*

Table 2.3 Place of death in England and Wales by age and sex, 1999

	NHS hospitals[1] and communal establishments (inc. nursing homes)		Non-NHS hospitals[2] and communal establishments (inc. private nursing homes)		Other[3] communal establishments (inc. aged person accommodation)		Hospice[4]		At home[5]	
	M	F	M	F	M	F	M	F	M	F
Aged 65 years and over	119 735	131 647	18 483	38 837	11 760	33 698	8373	7753	43 219	38 866
Aged 85 years and over	28 679	52 356	8199	25 127	6375	24 755	893	1124	7201	11 876

[1] NHS hospitals and communal establishments for the care of the sick does not cover NHS psychiatric hospitals but includes: *nursing homes*, general hospitals, sanatoria, geriatric hospitals and units, establishments for the chronic sick, mental hostels, homes or hostels for the mentally handicapped, maternity hospitals, and multifunction sites such as large hospitals.

[2] Non-NHS hospitals and communal establishments for the care of the sick does not cover non-NHS psychiatric hospitals but includes: *private nursing homes (including those for the aged)*, general hospitals, establishments for the geriatric and chronic sick, homes or hostels for the mentally handicapped, maternity hospitals, military hospitals, and multifunction sites such as large hospitals.

[3] Other communal establishments—schools for the mentally retarded and subnormal, holiday homes and hostels, common lodging houses, *aged persons accommodation*, assessment centres, schools, homes for the disabled or handicapped, rehabilitation centres, convents and monasteries, nursing homes, university and college hostels and halls of residence, approved schools, borstals and custody centres, detention centres, prisons, remand homes, YMCA, and YWCA hostels.

[4] Includes: Sue Ryder Homes, Marie Curie Centres, oncology centres, voluntary hospice units, and palliative care centres.

[5] Includes: those at the usual residence of the deceased (according to the informant), where this is not a communal establishment.

Source: Mortality Statistics: General (1999) England and Wales DH1 No. 32 ISSN 1469–2805, pp. 78–9.

staff are appropriate to the assessed needs of the service users, the size, layout, and purpose of the home at all times' and propose that at least 50 per cent of care staff should be trained to National Vocational Qualification (NVQ) Level 2 or equivalent by 2005 (excluding staff who are registered nurses) and that registration will mean that staff induction, training, and supervision arrangements are put into practice (DoH 2001a, Standards 27, 28, 36).

But what do we know about staffing? It was not until the Independent Sector Workforce Survey 1996 from the Local Government Management Board that we began to get more of a picture of independent sector provision (Local Government Management Board 1997). Based on a sample of 2791 private and voluntary homes (73 165 registered beds), this was the first comprehensive account of this workforce and it provided information concerning residential care homes, nursing homes, and dual-registered homes for a range of groups, the majority being for older people. The survey estimated that 74.1 per cent of staff were nursing and care staff and 23.4 per cent had support roles—cooks, cleaners, gardeners, and administrative staff. Only half of nursing and care staff worked full-time; a majority in all sectors and types of home were women with the proportion of male staff highest among managers and supervisors. The research also showed that 19.2 per cent of staff had worked in the home for less than a year and that this was higher in privately run homes than voluntary homes. The turnover rate was highest in dual-registered homes and the vacancy levels were highest for nursing staff who proved difficult to recruit.

In terms of training, not surprisingly, the proportion with qualifications was higher in nursing homes and amongst managers. In all sectors a small proportion of staff were studying for nursing qualifications or NVQs; some had reached NVQ assessor status. Unsurprisingly, training needs were identified in many homes. In a recent study of the skills and competencies of care assistants working with older people, Dalley and Denniss (2001) report findings from 418 surveyed care homes from all sectors of provision where 13 204 staff were employed of which 61 per cent were care assistants. The minimum wage was introduced in April 1999 at £3.60 per hour and in these homes the average for all homes was £3.88 per hour with local authority homes being part of a national local wage agreement offering around £4.50 per hour. In Chapter 8, we return to the training needs of care staff—suffice to say that in the main they are low-paid staff with little incentive to develop their employment potential.

The settings

The internal environment of care homes has changed over the years from the Victorian workhouses to the institutional settings that Townsend described, to adapted domestic houses used for nursing homes and care homes often enlarged through the addition of a modern extension to the group-living homes of the 1980s which tried to re-create the family group to newly built extra-care facilities (Peace *et al.* 1982; Willcocks *et al.* 1986; Peace 2002). To some degree all of these building types still exist. They have all been buildings that have combined public and private spaces for residents and staff to coexist. The working and living and dying environments have all 'rubbed shoulders' alongside each other, and the design of space can affect behaviour.

Patterns of staffing, needs of residents, and the impact of collectivity all have a bearing on how the daily routines of care homes have evolved. Issues of privacy and enabling older people to master their own personal space have been slow to legitimize. But there has been a growing recognition that in moving to collective care older people have a right to bed-sitting space that is adequate for personalization if so desired. However, the tension surrounding the cost of space remains for whereas improved environmental standards are now expected within newly built homes, these adaptations will no longer be required within existing premises (DoH 2001*a*, DoH 2003).

Of course another determinant of the capacity to obtain privacy is the opportunity to have a bed-sitting room of your own and the facilities it contains. Consequently the single-room ratio and the proportion of rooms with en-suite WCs have become markers of standards of amenity. Since the 1980s both of these trends have been developing and Laing (2002) shows that whereas in the late 1980s more than 50 per cent of rooms in for-profit nursing homes for older people were for more than one person and less than 20 per cent of rooms had en-suite WCs; by 2001 almost 80 per cent of rooms were single and en-suite WCs were provided in nearly 50 per cent of bed spaces. Of course there is variation between homes and the lack of shared facilities and provision of en-suite WCs is more common in for-profit nursing and dual-registered homes than residential care homes.

Regulation emerges and evolves

But who has been concerned with the quality and standards of such homes? Throughout the last century the reporting of poor practice and stark conditions led to the development of regulation through registration and inspection. This system began with private and voluntary sector provision moving at a much later stage to the public sector (Department of Health and Welsh Office 1990).

The Nursing Homes Registration Act, 1927 was the first statute to set down the now familiar procedures for registration: application accompanied by a fee; reasons for refusing registration; certification; cancellation of registration;

bye-laws concerning record keeping and notification of deaths, and the power to inspect (Abel-Smith 1964; Department of Health and Welsh Office 1990; HMSO 1990). This legislation also provided the first definition of 'nursing home' and 'maternity home' to appear on the statute:

> 'Nursing home' means any premises used or intended to be used for the reception of and the providing of nursing for persons suffering from any sickness, injury, or infirmity, ...
>
> (Nursing Homes Registration Act 1927: Section 10)

As Fig. 2.2 shows this early legislation was amended over the years giving both central and local government powers over the conduct of and facilities and services provided by nursing homes. Not-for-profit homes run by the voluntary sector were brought into the regulatory system in 1963 and the regulation of nursing and mental nursing homes were brought together in 1975.

The Nursing Homes Act 1975 delegated power for registration and inspection first to Area Health Authorities and later to District Health Authorities. Further legislative amendments followed and the types of regulated premises, including those offering medical and surgical services, expanded. Amendments made to the Nursing Homes Act 1975 and the Health Services Act of 1980 also related— for the first time—to the qualifications and residency of the 'person-in-charge' of the home and the level and qualification of nursing staff. All nursing homes had to be in the charge of either a registered medical practitioner, or qualified nurse, or in the case of maternity homes a certified midwife. The Health Circular HC(81)8 outlined that where a nurse was in charge of a home, they had to be a registered nurse and health authorities were able to determine staffing levels given the number and types of patients within particular homes.

Whilst they can be viewed in parallel the regulation of residential care homes followed a slightly different path. The 1948 National Assistance Act gave local authorities powers to arrange for the provision of accommodation within premises maintained by voluntary organizations (Section 26) and in 1968 this arrangement was extended to private sector homes (Section 44 Health Services and Public Health Act 1968). The first statutory requirement to regulate a private or voluntary home for people who were disabled or aged by a local authority was set out in Section 37–40 of the 1948 National Assistance Act and dealt mainly with registration being tied to what became commonly known as the fit person, fit building, and fit conduct of the home (Townsend 1962). Regulations concerning the 'Conduct of Homes' were not issued until 1962 and whilst covering a wide range of issues concerning health and medication did not comment specifically on practice for dying and death other than notification (Department of Health and Welsh Office 1990).

	Residential care homes	Nursing homes
Governing Acts	Public Health Act 1936 National Assistance Act 1948 Mental Health Act 1959 Residential Homes Act 1980	Nursing Homes Registration Act 1927 Public Health Act 1936 Nursing Homes Act 1963 Mental Health Act 1959 (beginning of regulation of mental nursing homes)
		Nursing Homes Act 1975 Health Service Act 1980
	Health and Social Services and Social Security Adjudications Act 1983	
		Health and Social Servics and Social Security Adjudications Act 1983 (did not repeat all legislation concerning nursing homes and mental nursing homes as it did for residential care homes)
	Registered Homes Act 1984	
	Children Act 1989	
	NHS and Community Care Act 1980	
	Registered Homes (Amendment) Act 1991	
	Care Standards Act 2000 (setting up of National Care Standards Commission and National Minimum Standards)	
Regulations	National Assistance Act (Registration of Homes) Regulations 1949	Nursing Homes and Medical Nursing Homes Regulations 1981
		Amended and replaced by:
	National Assistance Act (Conduct of Homes) Regulations 1962	Nursing Homes and Mental Nursing Homes Regulations 1984
	Amended and replaced by: Residential Care Homes Regulations 1984	
	National Care Standards Commission (Registration) Regulations 2001	
Codes of Practice	*Home Life* (Centre for policy on Ageing, 1984)	*Registration and Inspection of Nursing Homes: A Handbook for Health Authorities* (National Association of Health Authorities, 1985)
Standards	*Care Homes for Older People: National Minimum Standards* (DoH, 2001)	

Fig. 2.2 Legislation and documentation forming the basis of the regulation of residential care homes and nursing homes in England and Wales.

Source: based on Peace *et al.*, Re-evaluating Residential Care. Open University Press, p. 100; Dalley *et al.*, 2002, p. 108.

The 1960s, 1970s, and early 1980s saw growing concern over the quality of life provided for a variety of residents in care settings (Townsend 1962; Miller and Gywnne 1972; Kings Fund Centre 1980; Booth 1985; Willcocks *et al.* 1986) and a greater understanding of the impact of institutionalization on individual lives (Goffman 1961; Foucault 1977). Important research took place and of particular interest and influence were a series of publications arising out of the Residential Care Working Group of the Personal Social Service Council (PSSC 1977) which saw a need to develop further the function of registering authorities. Legislation and influential policy documents led to debate concerning the nursing care of older people living in residential homes and the need for a code of practice to improve the quality of care (DHSS and Welsh Office 1982).

The Health and Social Services and Social Security Adjudications Act 1983 (the HASSASSA Act) saw the development of *dual registration*. This was a recognition that there were residential homes where some residents required nursing care and others who only required residential care without the nursing component. The Act required that some homes providing both types of care should be registered with both District Health Authorities as nursing homes and with local social services authorities as residential care homes. These early developments in regulation culminated in The Registered Homes Act 1984 which began to develop a more systematic form of regulation for the growing independent sector of residential and nursing home provision.

Initially local authority based registration and inspection officers were called upon to develop tests of fitness for owners, managers, environments, and plans for care, and alongside these developments came accompanying guidance through the codes of practice: *Home Life* which covered older people and other vulnerable groups was developed at the Centre for Policy on Ageing (CPA 1984) and the *Registration and Inspection of Nursing Homes* (NAHA(T) 1985; 1988) by the National Association of Health Authorities and Trusts.

Over time both local authority provision and small homes with less than four residents became regulated (Peace *et al.* 1997) but during the 1990s the quality of care and the current system of regulation came to be questioned (Burgner 1996). The Burgner Report called for the development of national standards for care homes to overcome acknowledged inconsistencies within regulatory procedures. Since 1997, with the election of a New Labour government, a great deal of policy change has been introduced. In 1998, a white paper *Modernising Social Services* (DoH 1998) endorsed ideas surrounding changes to the system of regulation legislated through the Care Standards Act 2000. National Minimum Standards have been developed for a range of services currently regulated in England through the National Care

Standards Commission to become part of the Commission for Social Care Inspection. In England, the national minimum standards for care homes for older people were originally outlined in a consultation document *Fit for the Future* (DoH 1999) also developed through the Centre for Policy on Ageing and these were finally published in 2001 (DoH 2001a). In addition devolution of responsibility to the nations of the United Kingdom have seen the development of slightly different systems. For example, the Regulation of Care (Scotland) Act 2001 transferred powers and duties from local authorities to the Scottish Commission for the Regulation of Care.

Guidance on dying and death in care homes

With the development of these codes of practice and national minimum standards the issues of dying and death have been recognized alongside a great deal of information that is given regarding the development of a better quality of life. *Home Life* allocated a small section to the topic recognizing that those running residential care homes needed to identify whether they would be providing care until death and that if this was the case, their staff would need to develop necessary skills and communicate with outside experts:

> The importance of obtaining proper support from the community nursing services, the GP and, if necessary, specialists such as a visiting hospice nurse, cannot be over-emphasised.
>
> (CPA 1984, Section 2.7.5)

They emphasized that residents should feel secure within their care home and within their own room without the anxiety that they may be moved unnecessarily either internally or externally. Obviously, if a resident had requested specialist care such as within a hospice then these wishes should be followed. *Home Life* proposed that residents should be able to talk about their feelings and discuss requests concerning their end-of-life care such as relationships with family, friends, and religious staff. There was concern for informing relatives and enabling people to stay in the home if need be, and that records should be kept of any specific details concerning wills or property issues.

Alongside concerns for the residents, *Home Life* also considered the position of the staff recommending that they should understand the procedures to be followed when a death occurs and how they should be able to tell the other residents. They saw that there was a need for staff to understand local and cultural customs, and preferences of the deceased person and her family. But also *Home Life* recognized that this would be a time of stress for the staff and that they would need support, possibly from outside the home.

The documents provided by NAHA(T) (1985, 1988) gave little guidance concerning practice at times of dying and death in nursing homes.

Dying and death

68 When a home has admitted a resident with an assurance of 'care till death', the use of external sources of care, such as community nursing, or hospice service, is strongly recommended.

69 Intensive or terminal care should be given in a resident's own room and not in any special unit.

70 If a resident is aware he is dying, he should be consulted about his wishes on terminal care and funeral or cremation arrangements.

71 Contact should be made, if the resident wishes it, with the appropriate minister of religion.

72 When a resident is dying, the need for support to relatives, staff, and other residents should be recognized and met.

73 Local, cultural, and religious customs surrounding the death of a resident should be observed.

74 Proprietors should ascertain at an early stage who will take responsibility for a resident's property pending the proving of a will.

Checklist of recommendations from *Home Life*—(1984) CPA, p. 66/67.

Consideration is given to notification of deaths and the special needs of older people and people determined as terminally ill. While comment concerning older people centres on aspects of daily living from accommodation to occupation and leisure, that relating to the needs of the terminally ill makes this observation:

> Care for the terminally ill is not, however, restricted to hospices. All types of nursing homes need to be aware of the special needs of the dying...
>
> Staff need to consider both the physical needs and the emotional and spiritual problems of both the patient and the family. The use of pain control techniques and a consideration of the patient's individuality are necessary.
>
> (NAHAT 1985: 121)

As codes of practice were being developed for regulators, research and practice within residential care for all client groups was also brought together within the Wagner Report and published as *Residential Care: A Positive Choice* (NISW 1988*a*,*b*). However, it is interesting that neither the two volumes of the Wagner Report including the review of research (Sinclair *et al.* 1988) nor the report of the Wagner Development Group (NISW 1993) mention issues of dying and death within their discussion of residential living for older people. Only the subgroup reporting on 'Black Perspectives on Residential Care' considers

Announcing a death

News of a resident's death should be announced in a dignified and gentle way. It may be best to announce it quietly to individuals or staff groups to begin with but some more public announcement may also be appropriate in due course. Some people may find this public recognition comforting. It should never be assumed that people with dementia do not understand when someone has died. Some of the following possibilities might be appropriate:

- a minute's silence at an appropriate time;
- a photograph or some other personal tribute in a suitable place;
- opportunity to visit the dead person and pay last respects;
- a memorial or thanksgiving service or some other religious or cultural ceremony;
- lighting a candle;
- playing a favourite piece of music or reading a poem;
- a plant, picture or piece of furniture in memory of the person.

Plaques should be kept discreet so that the home is not overrun with Memorials.

From CPA (1996) *A Better Home Life*, p. 120.

issues of shared faith and spiritual experience in developing the culture within homes (NISW 1993: 68–85).

During the early 1990s, members of the CPA decided to revise the code of practice, *Home Life*. Whilst they still had confidence in that document, the circumstances of long term care for older people had changed. The NHS and Community Care Act 1990 had altered the way in which care was assessed, managed, and financed, and recognition of the growing numbers of older people living with dementing illnesses and the spectrum of accommodation and care found in sheltered housing, residential care homes, and nursing homes, led to a focus on the needs of these groups within a new code of practice.

In recognizing change the new publication *A Better Home Life* was able to focus in far more detail on issues of dying and death (CPA 1996). There was a recognition here—perhaps for the first time—that the culture of care surrounding living that had been the focus of attention for so long could now encompass dying and death. A whole chapter of the code was devoted to this topic and careful consideration was given to policies and procedures that would be able to recognize the wishes of the individual resident and allow for some non-intrusive planning to be made so that information concerning financial affairs, living wills, advance directives, and instructions for next of kin could be gathered. The period of dying was discussed looking at care and comfort and the use of external professionals; the situation of the resident within the home, and the involvement of relatives, other residents, and staff. The procedures to be carried out when someone has died are also considered by looking at how a death may be announced or recognized; what might happen regarding a funeral and how bereavement may touch many people. In this code the boundary between life and death is overcome and valued.

New developments

More recently it is hoped that research, policy, and practice will merge as regulators now work with National Minimum Standards when assessing the quality of care that is provided within care homes.

Death and dying

Outcome

Service users are assured that at the time of their death, staff will treat them and their family with care, sensitivity, and respect.

Standard 11

11.1 Care and comfort are given to service users who are dying, their death is handled with dignity and propriety, and their spiritual needs, rites, and functions observed.

11.2 Care staff make every effort to ensure that the service user receives appropriate attention and pain relief.

11.3 The service user's wishes concerning terminal care and arrangements after death are discussed and carried out.

11.4 The service user's family and friends are involved (if that is what the service user wants) in planning for and dealing with increasing infirmity, terminal illness, and death.

11.5 The privacy and dignity of the service user who is dying are maintained at all times.

11.6 Service users are able to spend their final days in their own rooms, surrounded by their personal belongings, unless there are strong medical reasons to prevent this.

11.7 The registered person ensures that staff and service users who wish to offer comfort to a service user who is dying are enabled and supported to do so.

Death and dying *(continued)*

11.8 Palliative care, practical assistance and advice, and bereavement counselling are provided by trained professionals/specialist agencies if the service user wishes.

11.9 The changing needs of service users with deteriorating conditions or dementia—for personal support or technical aids—are reviewed and met swiftly to ensure the individual retains maximum control.

11.10 Relatives and friends of a service user who is dying are able to stay with him/her, unless the service user makes it clear that he or she does not want them to, for as long as they wish.

11.11 The body of a service user who has died is handled with dignity, and time is allowed for family and friends to pay their respects.

11.12 Policies and procedures for handling dying and death are in place and observed by staff.

DoH (2001a) *Care Homes for Older People*, National Minimum Standards, p. 13.

As noted earlier, the new standards were initially developed by the CPA and the final standard on dying and death reflects the more well developed code of practice outlined above in *A Better Home Life*. Standard 11 is given above and a comparison of the two documents allows us to move from standard to practice.

Alongside this guidance we also have a *National Service Framework for Older People* (DoH 2001b) where person-centred care is acknowledged as an essential standard. Here attention is given to the behaviour of staff during end-of-life care:

> Supportive and palliative care aims to promote both physical and psycho-social well-being. All those providing health and social care, who have contact with older people with chronic conditions or who are approaching the end of their lives may need to provide supportive and palliative care.
>
> (DoH 2001b: 25)

They outline the main facets of this type of care as listed in the box opposite.

Future research will need to monitor the reality of the application of these standards. Nevertheless the quality of the time that residents spend within a care home still very much depends on the culture of care and the relationship developed between residents and staff.

Dignity in end-of-life care

Information and communication

- to facilitate choice about treatments and care options for older people and their carers
- control of pain and other distressing symptoms
- to anticipate, recognize and treat pain and distressing symptoms, and provide timely access to appropriate specialist teams, equipment or aids. There is evidence that older people are less likely to receive proper pain management.

Rehabilitation and support as health declines

- to ensure that quality of life and independence is maximized, and that an older person can remain at home (if that is their wish) until death or for as long as possible, through providing therapy and personal care and housing related support services.

Social care

- to maintain access to safe and accessible living environments, practical help, income maintenance, social networks, and information.

Spiritual care

- to recognize and meet spiritual and emotional needs through the availability of pastoral or spiritual carers reflecting the faiths of the local population.

Complementary therapies

- to provide evidence-based complementary therapies that support emotional, psychological, and spiritual well-being and help with symptom control.

Psychological care

- to anticipate, recognize, and treat any psychological distress experienced by the older person, carer, and their family.

Bereavement support

- to ensure the needs of family, friends, and carers are provided for, relieving distress, meeting spiritual needs, and offering bereavement counselling.

DoH (2001b) *National Service Framework for Older People*, p. 26.

An evolving culture of care

In setting the scene for the discussion of end-of-life care this chapter has reviewed the historical development of nursing homes and residential care homes showing how a concern over ways of living in frail old age has over-shadowed the issues of dying while living which are only just beginning to emerge as important. It is true that the conditions of collective living and poverty gave rise to a fear and loathing of care homes that permeated popular consciousness for much of the twentieth century and some would say beyond:

> What we also 'know', but, it may be argued, generally choose not to know, is that a silence persists, about the essence of residential living—a silence on the part of those older people who never enter residential care, but for whom the institutional option casts a shadow of deep anxiety and uncertainty in later life, as they fear its imminence; and a silence on the part of those who do actually cross the threshold into care.
>
> (Peace *et al.* 1997: 4).

The question is 'has this changed?' Older people living in care homes may lack some of the social capital of those living within their own homes but the difference continues to evolve. Living *en masse* has often led to a form of living managed for the organization rather than the person and the pressures of institutionalization. Consequently ageism and neglect have had to be faced before acknowledging individual need. As we have noted researchers over time have recognized the 'social death' of institutional care where residents have been seen as 'less than whole persons' and have sought to define accommodation and care that older people may value. In doing this they have failed to confront the experience of dying and death (Sinclair 1988; Peace *et al.* 1997). Will there be a change to a philosophy which understands that the existence of each resident is recognized through their life and their death. This concern forms the basis of this book and was recognized in *A Better Home Life:*

> As important to residents as the quality of their lives while they are living in the home will be the way in which they are cared for during the process of dying.
>
> (CPA 1996: 113)

To move us forward we therefore need to know more about who dies in care homes and begin to understand more about the people involved and those things that are important to them.

References

Abel-Smith, B. (1964) *The Hospitals 1800–1948*. Heinemann, London.

Bajekal, M. (2002) *Health Survey for England 2000: Characteristics of Care Homes and their Residents*. The Stationery Office, London.

Bauer, E.J. (1996) Transitions from home to nursing home in a capitated long term care program: The role of individual support systems. *Health Services Research*, **31**(3), 309–26.

Bebbington, A., Brown, P., Darton, R., and Netton, A. (1996) *Survey of Admissions to Residential and Nursing Homes for Elderly People*, DP 1222. PSSRU, University of Kent.

Booth, T. (1985) *Home Truths: Old People's Homes and the Outcome of Care*. Gower Publishing Co, Aldershot, Hants.

Brown, P., Bebbington, A., Darton, R., and Netton, A. (1997) *Survey of Admissions to Residential Local Authority Feedback: Summary Report to Cheshire Social Services Department*. PSSRU, University of Kent.

Burgner, T. (1996) *The Regulations and Inspection of Social Services*. HMSO, London.

Centre for Policy on Ageing (1984) *Home Life: A Code of Practice for Residential Care*. Report of a Working Party sponsored by the Department of Health and Social Security. Centre for Policy on Ageing, London.

Centre for Policy on Ageing (1996) *A Better Home Life*. Centre for Policy on Ageing, London.

Dalley, G. and Denniss, M. (2001) *Trained to Care? Investigating the Skills and Competencies of Care Assistants in Home for Older People*. Centre for Policy on Ageing Report No. 28. Centre for Policy on Ageing, London.

Dalley, G., Gearing, B., Peace, S. (2002) *Unit 20: Regulating for Quality. Workbook S: Rights, Risks and Control* from Open University Course: K202 Care, Welfare and Community. Open University, Buckingham.

Department of Health (1998) *Modernising Social Services: Promoting Independence, Improving Protection, Raising Standards, Cm 4169*. The Stationery Office, London.

Department of Health (1999) *Fit for the Future? National Required Standards for Residential and Nursing Homes for Older People*. DoH, London.

Department of Health (2001*a*) *Care Homes for Older People*. National Minimum Standards. The Stationery Office, London.

Department of Health (2001*b*) *National Service Framework for Older People*. Department of Health, London.

Department of Health (2002) *Guidance on the Single Assessment Process for Older People* HSC 2002/001: LAC (2002)1. Department of Health, London.

Department of Health (2003) Source: http://www.info.doh.gov.uk/doh/IntPress.nsf/page/2003–0070?OpenDocument

Department of Health and Social Security and Welsh Office (1982) *A Good Home*. A Consultative Document on the Registration System for Accommodation Registered under the Residential Homes Act 1980. HMSO, London.

Department of Health and Welsh Office (1990) *Making Sense of Inspection: A Training Course for Registration and Inspection Staff*. HMSO, London.

Foucault, M. (1977) *Discipline and Punish: The Birth of the Prison*, trans. Alan Sheridan. Allen Lane, London.

Goffman, E. (1961) *Asylums*. Penguin Books, London.

Higgs, P. and Victor, C. (1993) Institutional care and the life course, in S. Arber and M. Evandrou (eds) *Ageing, Independence and the Life Course*. Jessica Kingsley, London, 186–200.

Judge, K. (1986) Residential care for the elderly: Purposes and resources, in K. Judge and I. Sinclair (eds) *Residential Care for Elderly People*. HMSO, London.

Kings Fund Centre (1980) *An Ordinary Life*. Comprehensive locally-based residential services for mentally handicapped people. Project Paper No. 24. Kings Fund Centre, London.

Laing, W. (2002) *Healthcare Market Review 2001–2*. Laing and Buisson, London.

Levin, E., Moriarty, J., and Gorback, P. (1994) *Better for the Break*. HMSO, London.

Local Government Management Board (1997) *Independent Sector Workforce Study 1996*. LGMB, London.

Means, R. and Smith, R. (1983) From public assistance institutions to 'sunshine hotels': Changing state perceptions about residential care for elderly people, 1939–48. *Ageing and Society*, **3**(2), 157–81.

Miller, E.J. and Gwynne, G.V. (1972) *A Life Apart*. Tavistock Publications, London.

Ministry of Health (1926) *Report of Select Committee on Nursing Homes* (Registration). HMSO, London.

Ministry of Health (1949) *Twentieth Report of the Ministry of Health for 1938–9*, Cmd. 6089. HMSO, London.

Ministry of Health (1949) *Report of the Ministry of Health for the year ended 31 March 1948*, Cmd. 7734. HMSO, London.

Ministry of Health (1955) Ministry of Health Circular, 3/55. HMSO, London.

National Association of Health Authorities and Trusts (1985) *Registration and Inspection of Nursing Homes: A Handbook for Health Authorities*. NAHAT, Birmingham.

National Association of Health Authorities (1988) *The Registration and Inspection of Nursing Homes: A Handbook for Health Authorities*. Supplement NAHA, Birmingham.

National Institute for Social Work (1988a) *Residential Care: A Positive Choice*. HMSO, London.

National Institute for Social Work (1988b) *Residential Care: The Research Reviewed*. HMSO, London.

National Institute for Social Work (1993) *Residential Care: Positive Answer*. HMSO, London.

Netten, A., Darton, A., Bebbington, A., and Brown, P. (2001) Residential or nursing home care? The appropriateness of placement decisions. *Ageing and Society*, **21**(1), 3–24.

Nuffield Survey Committee (1947) *Old People, Report of a Survey Committee on the Problems of Ageing and the Care of Old People*, under the chairmanship of B. Seebohm Rowntree. Oxford University Press, London.

Office for National Statistics (2002) *Social Trends*. (2002 edition) The Stationery Office, London.

Peace, S. (2002) Block 2: People and Places from Open University Course: K100. *Understanding Health and Social Care*. Open University Press, Buckingham.

Peace, S.M., Kellaher, L. and Willcocks, D. (1982) *A Balanced Life? A Consumer Study of Residential Life in 100 Local Authority Old People's Homes*, Research Report No. 14. Survey Research Unit, Polytechnic of North London, London.

Peace, S.M., Kellaher, L.A., and Willcocks, D.M. (1997) *Re-evaluating Residential Care*. Open University Press, Buckingham.

Personal Social Service Council (1977) *Residential Care Reviewed: Report of the Residential Care Working Party*. PSSC, London.

The Royal Commission on Long Term Care (1999) *With Respect to Old Age*. (Cm 4192-L) The Stationery Office, London.

Sidell, M. (1995) *Health in Old Age*. Open University Press, Buckingham.

Sinclair, I. (1988) *Residential Care for Elderly People* in National Institute for Social Work (NISW) Residential Care: The Research Reviewed. HMSO, London, 241–91.

Sinclair, I., Stanforth, L., and O'Connor, P. (1988) Factors predicting admission of elderly people to local authority residential care. *British Journal of Social Work*, **18**, 251–88.

The Royal Commission on Long Term Care (1999) *With Respect to Old Age: Long Term Care—Rights and Responsibilities*. Cm 4192-I. The Stationery Office, London.

Thompson, P., Itzin, C., and Abendstern, M. (1990) *I don't feel old: Understanding the Experience of Later Life*. Oxford University Press, Oxford.

Townsend, P. (1962) *The Last Refuge*. Routledge and Kegan Paul, London.

Willcocks, D., Peace, S., and Kellaher, L. (1986) *Private Lives in Public Places*. Tavistock Publications, London.

Chapter 3

Who dies in care homes for older people?

Moyra Sidell and Carol Komaromy

Introduction

The answer to the question posed by the title of this chapter might seem self-evident but in fact it is rather complex. We contend that it has three major components. The first, 'who has died?' can be answered retrospectively with reference to mortality data. The second component, 'who is dying?' is much more difficult and hard to define. It raises many dilemmas both philosophical and practical and has important consequences for the care available to residents in care homes. A third question 'who will die?' lies in the realms of probability and is dependent on the ability to answer the first two. This chapter will concentrate on the first two questions. To address the first question 'who has died?' we draw on national mortality statistics as well as the quantitative retrospective evidence from Stage one of the OU Study (1) (see Chapter 1, p. 8) where we carried out a survey of 1000 residential, nursing, and dual-registered homes in three geographical areas of England—the North West, the West Midlands, and the South East. A postal questionnaire was sent to the registered managers of the sampled homes with a response rate of 41 per cent. Data were collected on home size, number of residents, numbers of staff, demographic details of the residents, number, and times of deaths, length of time spent as resident before death, and transfers to and from other institutions. In addition managers were asked to comment on training issues of staff relating to caring for dying residents. To address the more difficult second question 'who is dying?' we draw on the wealth of qualitative data from Stage two of the OU Study (1) and use case studies to draw out the complexities and implications inherent in this question (again see Chapter 1, p. 9).

Who has died in care homes?

A dramatic change in death rates took place over the twentieth century. Due to changes in life expectancy at the beginning of the twentieth century only

24 per cent of deaths were of people over 65; by the end of the century this had risen to 83 per cent (ONS 1999). The broader implications of this have already been discussed in Chapters 1 and 2. But the significance here is the fact that 18 per cent of these deaths now take place in care homes (Froggatt 2000). This amounts to about 32 000 deaths annually in these settings and this will probably rise given recent government policies aimed at moving older people out of hospitals and into care homes (DoH 1998, 2000).

The picture that emerged of who had died in the 412 care homes from Stage one of the OU Study (1) is presented in the following profile.

Profile of deaths in the surveyed homes

In the 12 months prior to answering the survey questionnaire (1995) there were 2180 deaths recorded in the 412 homes out of a total resident population of 10 035 people. On average this was a death rate of 22 per cent but this differed between the types of homes. Predictably the average death rate was higher in nursing homes at 36 per cent, and lower in residential homes at only 16 per cent with the rate in dual-registered homes being 23 per cent. This reflected the admission policies of the different types of homes at the time of the study. More physically frail and ill older people entered nursing homes than residential homes. As these distinctions become subject to placement decisions (see Chapter 2) we will only note differences between the types of homes where it is of particular interest.

Who died?

As Fig. 3.1 shows 53 per cent of deaths occurred in the over 85 age group with 33 per cent in the 75–85 age group and only 14 per cent amongst the under 75 year olds. The gender breakdown of deaths mirrored that of the resident population which was predominantly female with three times as many women

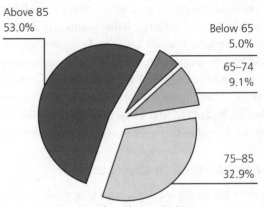

Fig. 3.1 Age at death.   Number of residents = 2180

as men in the surveyed homes. We were unable to derive any meaningful data on the ethnic origin of those who had died because the residential care population was predominantly white with only 1 per cent of all residents in the surveyed homes being from minority ethnic groups.

When did they die?

Predictably most deaths occurred in the winter months as Fig. 3.2 shows. This can put extra strain on staffing levels which might be depleted due to winter sickness.

The myth that most deaths occur at night was not entirely borne out by the data from OU Study (1) as Fig. 3.3 shows with just over half of deaths occurring in the daytime. However a significant number of deaths do occur at night and this too has implications for staffing levels which tend to be lower at night than during the day.

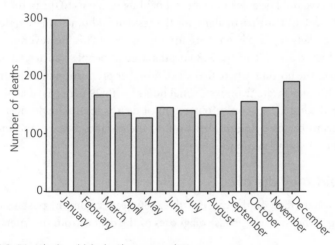

Fig. 3.2 Months in which deaths occurred.

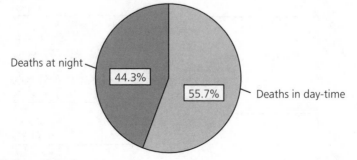

Fig. 3.3 Time of death.

How long had they been in the home before death?

Many of the residents had lived in the homes for a considerable length of time. This is clear from the data on the length of stay of the 2180 residents who had died in the 12 months prior to the survey. Figure 3.4 shows that 19 per cent of the people who had died had been living in the home for over five years with a further 29 per cent having been there for between two and five years. At the other end of the spectrum 18 per cent were relative newcomers having been in the home for less than three months and a further 8 per cent for between three and six months.

There were marked differences between types of homes with only 6 per cent of deaths in nursing homes occurring after five years as opposed to 28 per cent of residential home deaths. In dual-registered homes the figure was 22 per cent.

Because many of the residents had been in the home for a long time there was a strong sense that the home was indeed 'their home' and so it was important that they should be able to die there. Enabling residents to die in the home was an important issue particularly for the residential homes where residents were more likely to have been there for a long time. This, however, was not always achieved and 476 of the 2180 deaths were of people transferred out of the home to the hospital where they died. A higher proportion of those transferred to hospitals were from residential homes with 29 per cent of all deaths transferred compared to only 16 per cent of deaths in nursing homes. This issue of transferring dying residents out of the home is a vexed one and we discuss it more fully later in the chapter.

What did they die of?

We do not have data on the cause of the 2180 deaths from the postal survey and it was difficult to get precise diagnoses of the deaths from the interviews

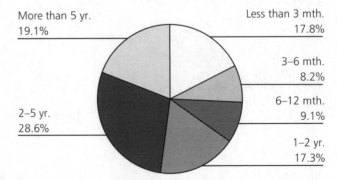

Fig. 3.4 Length of stay before death (all types of homes).

with registered managers of 100 homes from Stage two of the study. They gave the following broad categories. Deaths due to general deterioration was the commonest type of death described with death resulting from an acute episode such as a stroke or pneumonia being the next commonest. An actual terminal illness such as cancer or Parkinson's disease accounted for 15 per cent of the deaths described and only 9 per cent were described as 'sudden' and therefore unexpected. (Additional details are given in Chapter 11.)

The somewhat imprecise categorization of the cause of deaths made by the registered managers is emblematic of the difficulties that surround the second major question that this chapter addresses—the question of defining dying.

Defining dying

In order to understand how staff decided that someone was dying registered managers were asked to describe the process of dying of the last three residents who had died in the home in the previous six months (or more if no deaths had occurred for some time). They were encouraged to try to pinpoint at what stage they decided a resident was terminally ill and what actions this precipitated. As Table 3.1 illustrates most registered home managers defined the period of dying in weeks, rather than months, or longer.

Many registered managers noted that defining a resident as dying was particularly difficult prospectively. It was sometimes hard for them to identify an event which signalled the imminence of death particularly as they perceived many of their residents in a spiral of gradual decline with fluctuations in well-being over both short and long periods of time. Many registered managers expressed the sentiment, that people with chronic illness were likely to die at any time and commented that predicting timing and process was often difficult, with some residents dying quickly whilst more residents gradually deteriorated over a period of weeks.

Table 3.1 Lengths of period of dying—from Stage two retrospective accounts

	Total %
Sudden	9
Hours	6
Days	30
Weeks	40
Months	12
Years	3
$N = 133$	

There were a number of medical events which with hindsight, registered managers identified as the beginning of the downward spiral towards death. Residents who developed acute renal failure, chest infections or pneumonia or were losing consciousness were more likely to be defined as dying. These events were not always investigated because it was thought to be inappropriate to carry out invasive investigations in very old people. Registered home managers illustrated this point:

> She went off her feet for five days, she was bedridden and then everything just seemed to break down. She was confused, hot and sweaty, one minute and she had phases of going in and out of consciousness and she really was poorly.
>
> I went in one morning to get her up and she was not responsive and very lethargic, we thought she might have had a small CVA overnight; for the next two or three weeks she was bed bound, taking sips of water for about the first week and a small amount of diet but then did not eat or drink anything for about two weeks.

Sometimes death was thought to be precipitated by the residents and several managers held the view that once residents stopped 'helping themselves' they 'gave up' and this was a sign that they were about to die:

> She decided that she didn't want to eat anymore and as you gave her drinks she let them dribble out of her mouth . . . after a week they become so weak it is not fair to get them up, if they wish to die what are we fighting for, 75% of old people do decide that they want to die and they do.

The significance of defining dying

Although many deaths described by registered managers involved a very gradual deterioration they were keen to be able to recognize a point at which the resident could be described as dying. Staff also had duties of care to dying residents which were established either through written or unwritten routines, such as who should inform family and friends. When registered managers, and or GPs or other medical practitioners, defined someone as dying, it triggered a whole set of procedures of 'terminal' care and marked a significant moment which privileged care and resources for that resident. Without being awarded this status it was unlikely that residents would be afforded the same level of care, regardless of needs. Just what this care involved is the subject of the next chapter.

Another major implication of defining someone as dying was that they required more intensive or specialized care than was available in the home. When managers became aware that a resident was dying, the question of whether the resident should remain in the home or be transferred to another setting was often raised.

Transferring a resident to another setting

The issue of who to transfer, when, and under what conditions is a very complex one and one which exposes many contradictions. A qualitative study by Bottrell *et al.* (2001) identified some factors which influenced the decision to transfer residents to a hospital. These included the home's knowledge of the preferences of the resident and family; interactions with doctors; the home's technological and personnel resources and concerns about institutional liability. The OU Study (1) found similar influences although concerns about institutional liability were not so much in evidence and this could be due to the fact that the Bottrell study was conducted in America where litigation is more of a factor. However, as we noted earlier, the overwhelming view in most homes in the OU Study was a strong wish to keep the resident as long as possible, despite the extra burden that providing terminal care could place on the staff. The typical view expressed not only by registered managers but also care staff generally was that a crucial dimension of a dying resident's comfort related to remaining in what was now their own home, in familiar surroundings. The sentiment expressed by many respondents that 'this is their home' was closely related to the view that the resident had a right to die in the home:

> They are in the surroundings that they know, so we always keep them in their home, in their bedroom making sure there is music and flowers and just really making it almost pleasurable till the end.

But this 'home for life' philosophy to which most of the registered managers aspired did not always translate into practice and many residents were transferred to a hospital where they subsequently died. The ability of homes to provide terminal care was variable. Examples of problems in terminal care ranged from the administration of Morphine to residents unable to take oral analgesics to the need for surgery to relieve pressure pain caused by malignancy. Registered managers of some *residential* homes recognized that they were not able to care for people who needed more intensive nursing care and whose period of dying was likely to be longer than a few weeks. The manager of this voluntary *residential* home observed:

> If it looks as though it might be a short term nursing situation, then we wouldn't transfer them. If it looks as though, you know, within a couple of weeks they are going to get better or die, then they would stay here.

So defining dying and predicting death was a vital element in the decision to transfer a resident to a hospital. But heads of homes were usually dependent on the support of GPs to retain the dying person in the home:

> At the last stages the GP will say 'can you manage them here' and invariably we say 'yes', so they will die in this kind of environment rather than a hospital

environment, with people who know them, with people who understand most of their habits, likes and dislikes, so it will be with people who've shared their life experiences anyway. We invariably keep them here, not forcibly but if they want to. But we, the staff, are all committed to that.

Occasionally the GP would make the decision unilaterally as the registered manager of one voluntary *residential* home explained:

> . . . the doctor said, 'Having made the decision to ring me and bring me in, it is my decision now, and she should go into hospital.' So she went. She went at about two o'clock, and by half past six she was dead.

Those who did want to nurse residents until their death found that having to transfer someone out of the home because they were unable to manage the care created great dissatisfaction for them and their staff. The registered manager of a *residential* home described a very heavy resident who had deteriorated following an illness:

> She again was somebody who should have gone into a nursing home long before she did, but we knew that one transfer would kill her, which it did, going into hospital she died very quickly. We are reluctant to transfer people who are going possibly to succumb just because they are transferred, but then, they live longer than you expect every time.

This registered manager was not only expressing regret at not being able to care for someone until death, she was also presenting both the dilemma of whether to transfer someone, but also at what point it was best to do so. The following description of a decision by the registered manager of a small *residential* home highlights the commonly held belief that transfer to hospital hastens death. A 102-year-old resident suffered a haemorrhage and was thought to be dying. The registered manager managed to convince the GP that the resident should stay in the home to die. However, the resident did not die as predicted and was still alive a year later for which the registered manager offered this explanation:

> She is going to be 103 in June and the family were quite convinced she was going to die at Christmas, well actually we were all convinced. . . . So, you see, if you put people in hospital, they say, 'This is it, this is where I am going to die.'

This manager had worked out an explanation where the cause of death was partly due to the transfer itself, and she was not alone in this view. A lot of the registered managers who talked about this issue thought that the psychological effect of the home's 'rejection' of a resident contributed significantly to a resident's death following transfer. From talking to the majority of the registered managers it seemed that regrets associated with the transfer of residents out of homes involved both a frustrated desire to continue to care for residents until death and feelings of guilt that transfer may have in some way hastened death.

Although there was a general desire to keep dying residents in the homes to die, conflicts arose over whether or not a resident was dying, that is, defined as dying, and, if they were, whether they were in need of medical intervention which the home could not provide. The stated reasons for transferring people to hospital were medical conditions such as myocardial infarction, dehydration, cerebrovascular accident, and pneumonia—all of which they felt required more nursing care than they were able to give.

Many registered managers talked about the pressures they came under to transfer residents to hospital from relatives who, according to the registered managers, sometimes had unrealistic expectations about what could be done for their relative. As a registered manager explained:

> . . . I always tend to find that when the residents are asked what they want the majority of the time it is to be left here. It is normally the families that can't cope with the idea of the resident dying who will want to fight to the bitter end to keep them alive. They are the ones that want them shipping out.

The majority of the heads of homes said that, despite the pressure to 'do something', relatives were often relieved when residents could be nursed in the home until death, as this head of home explained:

> It is very hard to watch somebody not eating and drinking, you feel you should be doing something. . . . but her daughter and the doctor and myself discussed it. . . . The daughter did not want anything too strong done.

The decision to transfer a resident to hospital involved a negotiation with the GP and the relatives whose wishes were invariably adhered to:

> It is normally the relatives' decision whether they want them to go into hospital or not. If they say, 'No, leave her where she is that's fine' the GP normally abides by that.

Many GPs would advise against transfer because they thought that a hospital was the 'wrong place' for someone to die:

> Because I think you'd be subjected to all sorts of investigations and tests, and attempts at cure, which are not really wanted. . . . In my experience a lot of older people—they don't actively want to die, but they don't actively want to live either, and they certainly don't want drips and suction and antibiotics and goodness knows what. They just want to be looked after and kept comfortable.

The question of defining someone as dying creates many dilemmas and exposes many contradictions surrounding the decision to transfer a resident out of the home. The picture is very confused, if someone is defined as possibly dying but possibly treatable then arguments can be put forward for transferring them to a hospital where such treatment is available. However contrary arguments can also be mustered to keep them in the home to avoid the trauma of moving which might tip them over into death. If someone is said to be dying and not treatable then there is a strong argument for keeping them where they are because this is their home where they feel most comfortable. But the home must feel confident that they can provide all the care that is needed to keep them comfortable and if that is not the case then this can be an argument for transferring a dying resident where they can be looked after 'properly'. Add to these dilemmas the need to negotiate the decision with GPs and relatives then the stated wish of the home to maintain their residents till death becomes compromised.

Dying trajectories

The difficulty of this complex web of decision making is compounded by the problems of defining dying. We would argue that a more helpful way of addressing these issues of where and how best to provide terminal care is to operate with a notion of a *dying trajectory*. This would involve a much longer period of time than is usually envisaged by registered managers—typically a few days or maybe one or two weeks. In fact when asked about the cause of death heads of homes talked of general deterioration which for many residents had been taking place over a long period of time, months possibly years and for some it would probably date back to the admittance into the home. From her ethnographic study of life in a nursing home Sarah Forbes (2001) went so far as to say:

> Unfortunately, for many nursing home residents the chronic illness trajectory disguises the dying process, making it difficult to plan and provide end-of-life care. p. 39

Travis *et al.* (2001) suggested that most residents who are admitted on a permanent basis to care homes are in what they call a 'living–dying' state. They suggest that acknowledging this 'living–dying trajectory' has implications for care allowing for a blending of active treatment with palliative care. Figure 3.5 shows the appropriate treatment modalities at different stages of this 'living–dying trajectory'.

Here two case studies from OU Study (1) explore the dying trajectories of two residents described by the registered home managers.

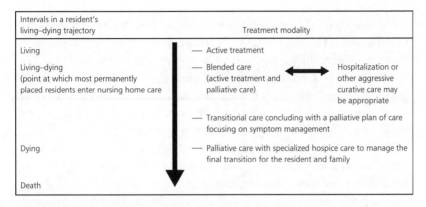

Intervals in a resident's living–dying trajectory	Treatment modality
Living	— Active treatment
Living–dying (point at which most permanently placed residents enter nursing home care	— Blended care (active treatment and palliative care) ⟷ Hospitalization or other aggressive curative care may be appropriate
	— Transitional care concluding with a palliative plan of care focusing on symptom management
Dying	— Palliative care with specialized hospice care to manage the final transition for the resident and family
Death	

Fig. 3.5 Living–dying care in long-term care.

Source: Travis *et al.* 2001: 154.

The death of Percival Walker

Percival Walker was a man in his mid-eighties, who was coping reasonably well at home after his wife died until he suffered a fall at home. He had lost consciousness briefly and was transferred to hospital. It was clear to the hospital staff that the main effect of the fall was that Percival had lost confidence. After three days, it was agreed that he should be transferred to The Pines care home for a one-month period of assessment. Percival settled into residential home life very well and after a month decided to stay there as a permanent resident. He made arrangements for his niece, his only close relative, to sell his home.

Percival had been an officer in the navy during the war and was delighted to meet a fellow resident called Charlie, who had also served in the navy, albeit as a seaman. They both reminisced about their Second World War experiences and exchanged accounts of various adventures.

At Christmas, when Percival had been in the home for six months, he suffered another fall when visiting the toilet during the night. The night-care assistant found him on the floor and got help by fetching Nasrin, the home-owner who lived in a flat within the home and was on call for emergencies. They returned him to bed and then Nasrin called the GP. Although Percival was very distressed he did not seem to have broken any bones and the GP decided to send him for an X-ray the next day, rather than make him go to the local Accident and Emergency Department as an emergency. This was arranged and Percival and the care assistant who accompanied him returned to the home later the next day with the news that there were no fractures.

Following this incident the home staff noticed that Percival was reluctant to move around as independently as he had done before the fall and over the next few months, he gradually withdrew from the life of the home. He needed to be coaxed into eating and even then would only eat small amounts of food. Although he and Charlie continued to sit next to each other in the dayroom, they did not talk in the animated way they had previously done, although they still exchanged pleasantries.

Percival had lost a lot of weight since his admission to the home and this, combined with his increasing reluctance to move made him at high risk of getting pressure sores. He complained of being uncomfortable and was occasionally incontinent. His GP visited him on a weekly basis and described his condition as one of 'gradual deterioration'.

One morning, when the care staff went to get Percival out of bed, it became clear that he had suffered a slight stroke. The GP visited and confirmed the staff's provisional diagnosis. She arranged for the practice community nurse to visit and to work out a plan of care for Percival. It was clear that he was deteriorating and in need of more nursing care.

Over the next few weeks Percival was nursed in bed. The staff had to do everything for him and they thought that he might be dying. They called his niece who stayed in a local hotel and visited every day. However, after a week Percival began to improve and the GP and community nurse agreed that the staff should begin to get him out of bed. Now that it seemed likely that he might recover the GP arranged for a physiotherapist to visit the home and assess Percival's condition with a view to helping him to become more mobile. Gradually, with support from external health professionals and the use of a wheelchair, Percival was able to get up and visit the dayroom each day. However he did not regain the use of his left side and continued to need a lot of nursing care.

Discussion

This type of trajectory is not unusual in dying older people. If this is applied to the trajectories in Fig. 3.5, it can be seen that at the point of admission to the home, Percival was at the 'living–dying' stage. There were several events that signalled a move into the 'dying' phase which, combined with his gradual deterioration, suggested that he was likely to die soon. Indeed, the home staff began to provide terminal care for him. This consisted of contacting his niece and instigating a care procedure that involved more intensive nursing care. Also the use of external professionals, the GP and community nurse, in terms of Fig 3.5 could be called 'blended care'. But, Percival did not die and this case serves to highlight the reality that many residents in care homes do not follow a trajectory of dying that is straightforward and continuously downward. The dying trajectory often consists of peaks and troughs and makes the terminal care management more complicated and difficult to predict. It seems that according to the suggested trajectory, the assumption of even a more complex downward spiral of dying cannot easily be planned for. Percival returned to the 'living–dying' status albeit lower on the trajectory than on admission.

The death of Miss Melanie Wilson

Miss Melanie Wilson was a single woman of 95, who was a retired teacher. She had lived in a small private care home, called The Meadows, for five years and stayed in her room most of the day, emerging only for meals and special events. She was a very private person and although she was well liked by the staff and got on well with most of them, she maintained a formal relationship with them and was addressed as Miss Wilson.

Miss Wilson was self-caring for most of her personal hygiene needs and had her own private bathroom. The staff helped her with an assisted bath twice a week in that someone helped her into and out of the bath. It gradually became apparent to the care staff that Miss Wilson was incontinent of urine and the registered manager, *Pauline* agreed to discuss this with her. She arranged for the community nurse to help her with her incontinence needs. The nurse agreed a strategy with Miss Wilson and supplied her with incontinence pads which helped her to cope.

As the weeks passed, Miss Wilson seemed to read less and also showed less interest in her hobby of knitting. She was often found asleep when staff came to take her to the dining room for her meals. She had always eaten quite well but she was clearly losing her appetite and eating much smaller amounts of food. She began to refuse her breakfast and preferred to stay in bed for most of the morning. Eventually she reached a stage where she would not get out of bed at all. *Pauline* grew increasingly concerned that the home staff could not manage her care needs and discussed the possibility of her longer-term future with the GP who suggested that Miss Wilson might be dying and asked the community nurse to visit to offer more support. It seemed likely that she was dying although no specific diagnosis was made.

The other home residents had missed Miss Wilson's presence at meal times and regularly asked after her. *Pauline* and the home staff told them that she was 'very poorly' and the staff discussed among themselves their belief that Miss Wilson was 'fading away' and had become 'tired of life'.

As Miss Wilson's decline continued the strain on the home staff became more acute. It was taking a considerable amount of time to care for her and they were worried that she might die at any time, but could not spare anyone to sit with her continuously. The home had just nine other residents and the care staff worried that they were neglecting them. The home employed only one care assistant at night and *Pauline*, who lived in the home, began to give more help with turning Miss Wilson at night. It was clear that the situation could not continue and *Pauline* asked the GP to try to arrange for her to be transferred out of the home. Although the GP tried to find a hospital bed for Miss Wilson, there was none available.

The situation continued for several weeks until Miss Wilson developed a severe chest infection. She deteriorated very slowly and began to refuse any drinks or medication in the form of antibiotics. The GP diagnosed pneumonia and it seemed that her death was imminent. She became unconscious after a further three days. Nevertheless it was not until five days later that she died. The staff felt drained by the experience of caring for Miss Wilson and unhappy that they might not have provided the specialist care that she seemed to need.

Discussion

Miss Wilson's decline and death followed a more straightforward dying trajectory than that of Percival. On admission to the home, she could be described as being close to the 'living–dying' status and she occupied this state for some time before she was formally categorized by the GP as 'dying'. However, it was not until the diagnosis of pneumonia and her unconscious state served as a marker of acute illness that Miss Wilson was considered to be close to death. The long-term chronicity of her condition and the long period of dying placed a serious strain on the ability of the home's staff to plan and manage her care. The example also highlights how difficult it is for staff in a small home to manage the care of dying residents alongside that of those who are deemed to be 'living'. This tension is a common feature of the OU Study (1).

What these case studies show is that, as an analytic tool, the representation described by Travis *et al.* (2001) is limited by several factors. First, the need to be able to categorize residents as actively dying and thus instigate palliative care is dependent upon a diagnosis of the status of dying. Even when there is an event that serves as a marker of the beginning of the stage of dying, this does not necessarily qualify as an accurate predictor of the imminence of death as the example of Percival shows. Second, the home's ability to call upon external support workers seems to be dependent upon a more robust marker of the beginning of the dying period, as in Miss Wilson's case and, even then, the support was quite limited. Third, the dying trajectory of people in homes is very different from those dying in hospices. And it must be remembered that care homes are not hospices and are not keen to be seen as primarily dying spaces. Making artificial distinctions between living and dying is the way homes cope with a situation which they see as otherwise too depressing for themselves and for their residents. But if they could operate with a longer notion of dying trajectories then the scope for applying palliative care in its broadest sense of relieving distress and discomfort would make much more sense and would be an appropriate approach to helping all residents who suffer from debilitating chronic illnesses. It should also help to avoid the sometimes unseemly and traumatic act of transferring someone out of the home at the point of death.

Conclusion

People rarely leave care homes except at death and the answers to the questions 'who has died' and 'who is dying in care homes' indicate that the distinction between living and dying in these settings is very blurred and sometimes transient. Yet the tendency has been to focus on the living aspects of the homes and deliberately play down the unpleasant fact of death and dying. The overall thesis of this book is that the palliative care approach has the potential to improve the quality of dying in homes. We would argue that if the notion of a longer dying trajectory were widely accepted then the palliative care approach could have much greater impact on the care available to all residents.

References

Bottrell, M.M., O'Sullivan, J.F. Robbis, M.A., Mitty, E.L., and Mezey, M.D. (2001) Transferring dying nursing home residents to the hospital: DON perspectives on the nurse's role in transfer decisions. *Geriatric Nursing*, **22**(6), 313–17.

Department of Health (1998) *Modernising Social Services*. The Stationery Office, London.

Department of Health (2000) *The NHS Plan: A Plan for Investment. A Plan for Reform*. Department of Health, London.

Forbes, S. (2001) This is Heaven's waiting room: End of life in one nursing home. *Journal of Gerontological Nursing*, November, 37–45.

Froggatt, K. (2000) *Palliative Care Education in Nursing Homes*. Macmillan Cancer Relief, London.

ONS (1999) *Office for National Statistics Annual Abstract of Statistics*. The Stationary Office, London.

Travis, S.S., Loving, G., McClanahan, F.I., and Bernard, M. (2001) Hospitalization patterns and palliation in the last year of life among residents in long-term care. *The Gerontologist*, **41**(2), 153–60.

Chapter 4

Managing dying residents

Jeanne Katz

Introduction

This chapter will examine how dying is managed in care homes in the United Kingdom and will build on issues raised in the previous chapter. The chapter begins with a short discussion of the philosophy apparent in care homes in relation to caring for dying residents and then explores current practice in care homes, focusing on some of the challenges facing managers. This is organized around the different components of palliative care. Case vignettes will illustrate the ways in which these deaths are managed. Finally features of what care staff believe constitute 'good' deaths will be described. Throughout the chapter comparisons and parallels will be drawn between the two main types of setting (nursing as opposed to residential).

Predicting dying in care homes is a complicated and complex task and one which home managers and care staff find difficult to do. Indeed defining dying in itself has a number of facets, not only practical but also philosophical. Homes that cater for the 'living' and indeed strive to rehabilitate frail people may be faced with the dilemma of defining dying without experiencing a sense of failure. This tension between caring for living as opposed to caring for dying residents may parallel the care/cure dichotomy which has been debated in medicine and nursing for the past 50 years. These discussions relate to the transition from attempting to cure the illness through medical interventions such as aggressive treatment to acknowledging that the person is not going to recover and requires nursing and/or social care. Therefore philosophical difficulties related to defining dying and indeed caring for dying residents in the care home sector may simply reflect some of those issues in the wider society.

Principles in caring for dying residents

Before exploring the care of dying people in care homes using a perspective derived from palliative care it is important to revisit the 'spirit' of palliative care. This might be summarized as understanding the pain and suffering of dying people, addressing their individual needs (person-centred care), ensuring that a whole person approach is used in planning end of life care and enabling dying people where possible to exercise choice and control over their care.

The first OU Study set out to explore the applicability of the principles and practices of palliative care to home settings. First of all it investigated whether or not home managers were familiar with the concepts of palliative care. Most carers, including home managers working in care homes did not recognize the different components of palliative care, nor were they committed to providing holistic care within that paradigm. Discussing the application of palliative care principles to home settings with the two-thirds of the 100 home managers who were not familiar with these was therefore inappropriate. Only 15 of the remaining 33 home managers who were familiar with hospice philosophy had a detailed understanding thereof (OU Study (1)). Previous contact with the Macmillan service or hospice care team in any capacity (professional or personal) increased managers' awareness of the potential specialist palliative care services could provide in relation to symptom control and emotional support. Yet few managers could see the relevance of specialist palliative care services beyond caring for someone with cancer. Only six of the 100 home managers interviewed who both understood palliative care and thought that it was highly relevant to their settings had made attempts to deliver something approaching palliative care to their terminally ill residents. The translation of good intentions into practice was less easy.

Chapter 2 demonstrated how care homes have their own philosophies and culture which accommodates caring for dying residents. Although few managers interviewed in OU Study (1) understood the specific principles and practices of palliative care, their conceptualization of good end-of-life care resembled some palliative care principles.

Descriptions of good end-of-life care encompassed the aim that dying residents should be secure, comfortable and pain free during their last days (Katz *et al.* 1999). This vision was comprised of three interrelated principles. The first was the ultimate goal that dying residents should be enabled to *die with dignity*. Physical deterioration and decline, such as bedsores, oedema, and immobility in themselves create a loss of dignity for older people (Hanson and Henderson 2000). It was therefore difficult to see how dignity could be maintained if it was something attributed to the ageing process. Yet home managers in the OU Study tended to define dying with dignity more in terms of '*treating the resident as a person till they died*' and enabling the dying person to '*appear to still be of use*'.

The second principle, discussed in the previous chapter, was that the home staff were committed to *retaining residents in their familiar surroundings* till death if at all possible. Despite the strength of their conviction that residents had the right to die in what had become their own home the operationalization of this intention depended on the type of home and staff's own perceived ability to 'nurse' the dying resident. *Residential* home managers were usually willing to keep residents in the home to die if they felt capable of providing the required hands-on care often with the support of the community nurses. On the other hand *nursing homes* saw themselves as able to provide intensive nursing care to dying residents.

The third principle (connected with the second) was that residents were entitled to *good pain control and nursing care*. This was by far the most important principle and therefore is the basis for much of the rest of this chapter which delineates the current practice in caring for dying residents.

Current practice in managing dying residents

Using the main components of palliative care we now explore the needs of dying residents using the information provided by OU Study (1) as illustrative of how dying people are managed currently in care homes.

Addressing dying residents' needs

Most care home residents experience pain and other symptoms and these need addressing regardless of whether the resident is defined as 'dying'. Forty to eighty per cent of nursing home residents experience pain—chronic conditions include low back pain, arthritis, and neuropathies (Forbes 2001; Fisher *et al.* 2002). Pain is also reported in major joints, legs, and feet (Helme and Gibson 2001).

In the terminal stage long term care residents suffer from the following symptoms according to frequency: pain, dyspnea, depression, anxiety, and loneliness (Baer and Hanson 2000); episodes of acute illness include pneumonia, sepsis, and dehydration (Hanson *et al.* 2002). Symptoms may change as death approaches—Hall *et al.* (2002) noted that during the last 48 h of residents' lives symptoms included pain, dyspnea, noisy breathing, delirium, dysphagia, fever and myoclonus. Dyspnea was the most common symptom, followed by pain and then noisy breathing.

Recognizing physical pain

Recognition and assessment of residents' pain and symptoms are clearly central to good management. Studies suggest that a significant number of older people do not receive sufficient pain management (Gagliese and Melzack 1997), especially those with cancer (Casarett *et al.* 2001). Doctors attending nursing homes often do not recognize pain as a difficulty nor prescribe adequate analgesia for residents (many studies reported by Miller *et al.* 2002). Over 25 per cent of residents who report pain receive *no* analgesia, and this percentage increases with cognitive impairment (cited in Fisher *et al.* 2002). Part of the problem relates to difficulties in assessing pain, and currently studies are underway exploring the use of different pain assessment scales with people residing in long-term care facilities in order to improve pain recognition by carers (e.g. Fisher *et al.* 2002).

Pain assessment and symptom control

As noted in Chapters 2 and 3 the majority of carers in long term care facilities in the United Kingdom and in other English speaking countries are low paid, untrained, or poorly trained women. These carers are most familiar with residents and should be sensitive to changes in residents' behaviour but their training rarely includes assessment of residents' levels of discomfort. Hanson and Henderson (2000) suggest that certified nursing assistants (the equivalent of care assistants in the United Kingdom) 'have a critical role in assessing the needs of a dying LTC facility resident, because they are often the first to observe symptoms of critical or terminal illness. Their observation of subtle changes in behaviour, mood, or intake that characterize terminal decline for frail residents are critical to good patient care' (p. 226).

But assessing pain is a complex task in older people and cognitive impairment can be a complicating factor for symptom management. Flacker *et al.*'s (2001) study in a nursing home demonstrated differences in pain assessment between nursing aides, qualified nurses and physicians, and noted that aides' perceptions of residents' pain was greater than either nurses or physicians. Engle *et al.* (2001) also noted that both licensed practical nurses and nursing assistants underestimated residents' pain frequency but that the latter were more accurate than the former in relation to pain intensity.

Twenty per cent of all managers in the OU Study (1) contended that residents should not have to die in pain and suffering; 25 per cent of nursing and dual-registered home managers highlighted poor or inadequate management of pain and symptoms in terminal care as a major problem. Despite the differences in staff skills, nursing home and residential home managers had similar views in relation to pain and symptom control.

There was a wide variation of ability and willingness within homes to respond to pain and symptom relief. Inability to control pain was for many *residential* homes one reason for considering admitting a resident to hospital. They saw controlling pain as the responsibility of outside health professionals, particularly community nurses and GPs. *Nursing* home managers too associated adequate pain control with regular visits and communication with GPs (similar to Maddocks and Parker 2001). The extent to which GPs in turn could provide good pain control and symptom relief partly depended upon their own specialist knowledge or willingness to call in specialist advice or services (see Chapter 7). Just over 10 per cent of all managers described inadequate or poor responses from the GP when someone was terminally ill particularly in relation to the need for better pain management.

Yet, some managers understood the principles of good pain management:

> I am a firm believer in pain relief. I know the principles of how morphine works and yes, it kills the pain and also represses your respiratory system. In the end it is very often that that kills you, but at least you are not in pain, and it's not an issue, you are not thinking 'are they (in pain) or aren't they?'

However, similar to the respondents in the studies reported by Maddocks and Parker (2001), managers in OU Study (1) maintained that it sometimes took an unacceptable time getting pain under control. Managers in both OU Studies reported that GPs disregarded their assessment of a resident's pain. Many examples of failure to control non-cancer related pain were reported and this has considerable implications for dying residents as most suffer from conditions other than cancer. For example, a resident complained about the pain from contractures following his stroke; despite valiant efforts the staff usually could not ease the pain. His wife explained:

> I knew he had pains in the leg and he used to cry out, you know. I knew he had cramp pains in the leg, but they said they were giving him medication for it.... He was obviously shouting in pain, you know and as he couldn't speak it was the only way he could express his self. There were two or three times when they gave him medication and I think it did help.

Carers reported that many GPs seemed reluctant to prescribe adequate analgesia for pain not associated with cancer:

> The last person who died with severe pain was the lady with arthritis, that sticks out in my mind because following that I have always argued in favour of people with arthritis having kind of hospice care and having treatment for pain. I remember back when it was time for this lady to be put on Morphine, which I think we did actually win in the end, but because, I think I was told at the time, because she didn't have cancer she couldn't have Morphine medication, which was to me crazy. The lady was dying, she was in a lot of pain.

However, in some cases the pain control was relatively simple and easily managed:

> She was just on paracetamol for pain. She was not in pain much, she was not particularly chesty or had problems breathing so we did not feel she need any hyoscine or anything like that. She was unable to take anything orally.

Syringe drivers are often the preferred route of administering analgesia to dying people who cannot cope with oral medication. Usually syringe drivers are placed on the resident's chest and facilitate effective and continuous flow of pain control. In OU Study (1) very few homes owned syringe drivers and were therefore dependent on outside sources to not only provide them but also service them. This included nursing homes with specified terminal care beds (Komaromy *et al.* 2000).

Managers (and specialist palliative carers) were concerned that access to syringe drivers was far from automatic and could be affected by local policy, the home's status, and the GPs' views about the suitability of this method of delivery of analgesia. One community nurse noted that patients dying at home were perceived to have higher priority over residents in care homes for access to the very limited number of syringe drivers in the area (Komaromy *et al.* 2000).

It is relevant to observe here that few homes, especially *residential* homes, called upon specialist palliative care support to help with pain and symptom control when a resident was believed to be in the terminal stage. A small percentage had on occasion used the services of a palliative care specialist, most commonly a Macmillan nurse or a member of the hospice team. A few *nursing* homes had registered terminal care beds and provided terminal care, including pain and symptom management with occasional input from a palliative care team member. The use of external professionals is discussed in detail in Chapter 7.

Physical symptoms other than pain

Home managers in OU Study (1) focused on physical pain as the main component of suffering and rarely mentioned other symptoms which were clearly present. For example, the research team observed residents who suffered from symptoms such as weakness, nausea, difficulty in breathing, and/or swallowing, as well as psychological distress and loneliness (Maddocks and Parker 2001; Hall *et al.* 2002). In Canada by auditing a pain and symptom chart Hall *et al.* (2002) found that 23 per cent of residents with dypsnea were not treated for this symptom; while 99 per cent of residents with pain received adequate medication only 37 per cent of residents with delirium were treated. In the OU Study very few managers described any of these symptoms. Indeed only one manager, that of a private *nursing* home raised constipation, a symptom routinely focused upon in palliative care, as a problem and she framed it in terms of 'physical pain'.

Not all symptoms noted in the OU Study were related to a particular medical condition. Some were a result of being in bed for a long period of time:

> ... she broke down poor soul, her shoulders, then her back went, her hips, and I mean poor soul, she had a hole in her back you could put your fist through and

she never moved. But you didn't know where to touch her to turn her and I think, well, if there's a god up there, why?

From exploring the nature of the physical conditions common in dying residents we now examine ways in which homes addressed these.

Components of good nursing care

'Tender loving care' was the phrase used by home managers as well as GPs in OU Study (1) to describe appropriate care for dying residents. Good end-of-life care usually related to their perceived ability to carry out 'nursing type procedures'. In OU Study (1) turning was a fundamental part of 'full nursing care'; 'good nursing care' included turning, oral care as well as ensuring general comfort.

'Turning' bed bound dying residents to prevent pressure sores was an overarching theme for most homes, regardless of region or designation. Preventing pressure sores was the criterion by which homes judged themselves in relation to providing good care.

> She was basically sort of just turned hourly, full nursing care for a week and a half until she died.

Regular turning also ensured frequent visits to dying residents, minimizing the risk of a resident lying dead for a lengthy period of time before being discovered. Only rarely did managers question the wisdom of turning a terminally ill person, for whom turning might create additional discomfort or acute pain.

Providing general comfort to residents was based on carers' personal relationships with residents (Hanson *et al.* 2002) and their vast experience of caring for older people with chronic, long-term conditions (Froggatt 2001). Carers in the OU Study (1) maintained that experience enabled them to perceive residents' requirements even when the resident was unable to articulate them. Nevertheless they usually undertook the following tasks:

> We did all the things we could, washed, fed, watered, turned her over, eased the pain, creamed her elbows, and creamed her heels.

Sometimes this required the support of community nurses. Heads of *residential* homes cited the pivotal role of community nurses in caring for dying residents, particularly in relation to setting up syringe drivers. In addition community nurses provided mattresses and many other useful devices for staff in residential homes. They were seen as an essential resource (this is discussed further in Chapter 7):

> The community nurse was involved because she was breaking down round the back area, that was regularly twice a day.

Impediments to good physical care

The process of providing physical care for dying residents depends on the physical layout of the homes, the culture as well as other factors covered elsewhere in this book. As noted in Chapter 2 many homes in the United Kingdom are not purpose built and may be converted from other institutions or private domestic lodgings. The physical plant of the homes in OU Study (1) were very diverse, some retained the basic original layout of a large, family home, others were modern and purpose built. The trend toward single room provision continues, and at the time of the survey in OU Study (1) there were only 11 per cent of the residents sharing rooms, of which 4 per cent were married couples.

Finding appropriate space to care for dying people that is accessible to all the services required by the dying person is not always straightforward. The size, layout and facilities of the bedroom influences the way in which care can be given to a dying resident as well as whether relatives can stay in the room. Hard work is involved in pulling a bed away from the wall, and bending down to lift a resident who may be difficult to move. Sluice and other facilities were not always conveniently located (Komaromy *et al.* 2000).

Attending to residents especially at night unavoidably leaves residents in other parts of the home unobserved and isolated. In OU Study (1) some homes were on several levels and involved staff walking a relatively long distance to respond to residents' calls. While the majority of the homes had a call system not all of the residents were able to use it and residents who were dying were often those least able to summon help.

In summary, like findings from Hanson *et al.*'s study (2002) carers in OU Study (1) saw the poverty of resources in the home as an important barrier to high quality care of dying residents.

Emotional needs of dying residents

> Death in a nursing home was often characterised by psychological suffering.
> (Hanson *et al.* 2002: 120)

Many studies have reported psychological and social suffering of home residents—these include loss of personhood, independence, and social contacts. Respondents in Hanson's study (2002) felt that residents needed 'individualised' care to compensate for their social isolation and psychological suffering. Respondents in the OU Study did not focus on individualized care to the same extent although they recognized some symptoms of psychological distress as well as physical symptoms, for example, 'restlessness' or 'agitation'.

Addressing the more obvious emotional needs of people residing in homes for older people is a complex task and depends very much on the assessment, anecdotally or otherwise of the mental capabilities of the residents. In OU Study (1) managers emphasized providing comfort and reassurance to dying residents—residents should be made to feel wanted, given time and energy, and most of all listened to.

Managers were unable to ascertain whether or not dying residents knew that they were dying yet they recognized that the dying resident may be afraid. In that case they attempted to ensure the resident wasn't left alone for long periods of time:

> Her key worker would come in and sit with her because she was very afraid. She was aware she was dying in her conscious times and she was frightened.

The question of sitting with a dying resident was contentious. About a quarter of respondents stated that they had a policy that residents should not die alone. Carers in the OU Study (1) often described themselves as the residents' surrogate family and some stayed past the end of their shifts to be with residents when they died (similar to Hanson *et al.* 2002). But it was evident from the accounts of managers, carers, and other informants that even when death was anticipated there were residents who died alone. Staff numbers and workloads did not permit staff to sit with residents particularly during busy periods in the home. This is particularly pertinent during the evening and even more so during the night when many homes had only two or three staff members on duty, each responsible for up to 10 residents each.

The staff resources that each home was able to marshal to enable a colleague to sit with a resident during the dying period varied between homes, as did their commitment to making this possible. Religious homes, most particularly Catholic homes, prioritized sitting with a dying resident and they strove to have someone present at the moment of death. One of the sisters or a priest would pray with a dying resident because in the Catholic faith, death is as significant an event as birth. Some homes attempted to ensure that a staff member sat with residents throughout the dying period whilst other homes were less able to do so, yet most agreed that at the moment of death it was important to have someone present:

> We do try if at all possible to be with them and there have been occasions when they have been on their own, but if at all possible we try and keep somebody with them, yes.

Some home managers disagreed with this, suggesting that it was enough for the staff to visit the resident very regularly:

> When someone is ill, well very poorly, we sit with them for periods of time, but not a sort of vigil. Well I don't think it's what they want, they need peace and quiet.

Another reason for ensuring that the resident did not die alone was that dying alone was perceived as distressing not only for the dying person but for those left behind:

> ... one of the biggest questions we are asked a lot is, 'Were they alone?' I think that is one of everybody's fears isn't it, that you die on your own. We find that a lot.

Several managers stated that they believed residents preferred to die on their own, and needed that privacy, even if it went against their own preferences:

> There was always somebody with Alec, going on for 10 weeks. Day and night there was someone. Then in the end, we all came to the conclusion that Alec's waiting for something. Or if he is going to die, he's going to die on his own. And then one afternoon he died ... on his own.

Social needs: Lonely dying

In contrast to Hockey (1990), OU Study (1) did not find that dying residents were consigned to a 'dying room', however it was clear that many dying residents were isolated as reported in other settings (Glaser and Strauss 1965). For example, one resident increasingly withdrew to his room over a period of months and this meant that finally his death seemed to pass unnoticed by the other residents in the same unit. Conversely, when residents were defined as dying in a large religious voluntary *residential* home the bedroom door was ajar to facilitate visits from staff and other residents. This and other religious homes were more open about death and dying than homes with no religious affiliation (Komaromy *et al.* 2000).

Dying in a shared room

Although dying alone was seen as undesirable, dying in a shared room was equally problematic. The need for privacy for the room-mate competed with needs of the family of the dying resident. There were also other disturbances to the room-mate both before and at the time of death.

Home staff explained that there were three options when a resident was dying in a shared room. First, the dying resident could be moved to a sick room which most managers considered inappropriate. The manager of a voluntary *nursing* home represented this minority view:

> We juggle the beds around and they go into a single room, because it's not fair that where especially with the amount of care they have, (you're going in and out day and night) and it will disturb the other person. At night the other person isn't going to want somebody else's family sitting in their room, so if we know someone is dying we will transfer them into a single room.

The manager of a local authority home noted that the old tradition of moving sick and dying residents to rooms near to the staff room had been stopped when they learned that the residents called this corridor 'death row' (similar to Maddocks and Parker 2001).

The second option was to move the room-mate to another room and although this practice was preferred to the former option it was also uncommon. This was because the decision to move residents was in part dependent upon the level of awareness of the non-dying resident:

> Well if they are in a shared room then obviously we get the other lady or gentleman to come and sit in the lounge or if we have another room we will put them in another room, or if there's someone in a single we would ask them if they would mind changing, just so they could be on their own, if not then we would have to get the other lady or gentleman up and make them as comfortable as we can in one of the lounges.

While the final option of leaving the residents in the same room was thought to be unsatisfactory it seemed to be what happened most often. During observations in a voluntary *residential* home, a resident was left in a shared room with her room-mate because she was thought to be unaware of what was happening. Despite the resident's apparent lack of awareness, the staff intended moving her out of the room if the death occurred at night.

Although most managers thought that sharing a room was undesirable, especially if a resident was terminally ill, a small minority noted the advantages of sharing a room:

> I know the new thing is the single rooms, everybody wants a single room, but we find here especially when it comes to them not feeling very well it is very comforting to have somebody else in the room with them.

Spiritual support

Although studies have found that residents dying in care homes might have emotional and social needs (e.g. Hanson *et al.* 2002), in OU Study (1), other than in homes with a religious affiliation (and all those in the sample were Christians), few managers explicitly acknowledged existential pain, although they recognized that residents could be frightened of dying.

Dying residents' attitudes towards death

In OU Study (1) care staff expressed their views about the attitudes of older people towards death. Managers, in particular, maintained that older people are 'philosophical' about the deaths of others and of self and suggested that some residents were tired of their lives and wanted to die. Managers often came to these conclusions intuitively, without consulting dying residents. Most were convinced that older residents are resigned to death but do not want to talk about it. Similar to Froggatt's (2000) findings in case studies of four nursing homes, many respondents in both OU Studies appeared to lack confidence in respect to talking with residents about death. (Very few carers had had any communication skills training.)

However a few managers reported speaking to residents about death. They did not find that older residents were universally philosophical, on the contrary they held a multiplicity of views. For example, residents dying in the 12 homes attached to a religious order were reportedly not afraid of death and willing to talk about it. Talking about death was seen by managers in these homes to have reduced the anxiety levels of all concerned as resident and often family were prepared and accepting of death. Even those managing homes not associated with religious orders noted that residents with spiritual beliefs seemed to be less anxious about death. This impression has been replicated in a study of about to be bereaved relatives of hospice patients (Walsh *et al.* 2002).

> People go out kicking and screaming because they don't know what's coming next and I find that people who have more of a simple faith, no matter what their beliefs are, tend to have an easier time.

The question of older people being more resigned to death has been vigorously debated in the literature (e.g. Moss and Moss 1996; Howarth 1998) and many research findings directly exploring the views of older people do not confirm the assumptions made by managers in OU Study (1). Forbes's study (2001) revealed that American nursing home residents described death as a common experience and for them death was the expected outcome of admission to a nursing home.

Ministers of religion

Most homes in OU Study (1) regularly called upon the services of ministers of religion. Sunday services were often conducted in homes which did not have their own chapel.

The ways in which ministers were used varied considerably between homes. Religious voluntary homes used formal religion both to prepare residents spiritually for death and for last sacraments. Non-affiliated homes called ministers of religion to residents who requested visits, but did not appear to address the spiritual needs of residents without a specific faith. Some homes used the minister for staff support when a resident died:

> ... and with Father Richard, who not only came to see Eileen, but to make sure that the staff were alright as well and were able to cope with it.

When residents were dying it was usually left to the family or the resident to make a request for someone to visit. One of the ministers who visited a voluntary *dual-registered* home suggested that he was regrettably under-used in that staff tended to send for him to perform religious tasks, like the sacrament of the sick when residents were very close to death. He preferred to be available to offer emotional and spiritual support around death before they neared death. He regretted not being used more in the counselling and supportive role for staff. A consequence of the way in which his services were used was to make his presence a signal to residents that death was imminent. He thought this deterred people even further from calling him into the home for less formal tasks. He felt that he was a valuable resource to the home and that the skills he had to offer were not used to the best advantage (Komaromy *et al.* 2000).

Conditions for good practical management of dying residents

In addition to findings from OU Study (1), others studies exploring the care of residents dying in care facilities suggest that supportive or palliative care is not delivered quickly enough to dying residents and that those managing their care act too slowly or indecisively (Travis *et al.* 2001). Homes in OU Study (1) that appeared to deliver good end-of-life care set up a care plan once a resident was defined as dying. The process of determining the necessity of a care plan and deciding how to divide the work was described by the manager of a Local Authority *residential* home:

> As someone deteriorates we set up a care plan that everybody needs to follow; the morning shift would discuss and say, ' Well I'll do the first hour' and then somebody else does the second, third and fourth and take it in turns, like I'll feed her today. . . it would be something that was up on the wall, that was agreed on the day because you might get somebody that doesn't particularly want to sit with them so you wouldn't say you have to, you know, you share it out between the ones that don't mind doing it. Of course nobody has said they don't ever want to, but you could quite easily come across a new member of staff, you couldn't expect to go and sit with somebody.

The complexity of care plans varied, from very basic observational remarks to collecting quite sophisticated information such as fluid balance measurements.

A very important factor that determined whether good end-of-life care could be delivered related to staffing—levels, quality, and training of staffing (OU Study (1)). Peace *et al.* (1997) note how changing needs of residents make workloads in care homes unpredictable. Depending on the nursing needs of a dying resident, this can create pressure for care home staff. Many homes in OU Study (1) reported over-stretched staff resources and difficulties in obtaining additional staff for a variety of reasons, one of which was financial. Particularly during the winter months when more residents die and staff succumb to sickness, staff shortages can impact considerably on the care of dying residents. At night the situation was even more grave—some homes that were split into units only had one carer on duty—this meant that if a dying resident in one unit needed turning, for example, residents on another unit would be unattended (Komaromy *et al.* 2000).

Some carers needed actual physical support to care for a dying resident: for example, help with actual business of caring, lifting, feeding, and delivering drugs to the dying person. Additionally, carers may need relief from their other duties for that shift if they are deployed to sit with the dying or deceased resident or their relatives. This means that even carers who have not necessarily been involved with the dying resident may have to carry out additional tasks. Many homes in OU Study (1) reported that carers stayed on past the end of their shifts to ensure continuity of care for dying residents—this obviously had implications for subsequent work rosters.

Lack of available staff means that even if managers intend to ensure a dying resident is not left alone (as was the intention of 60 per cent of managers interviewed in OU Study (1)), this is not possible as it would affect the normal routines of the home. However observations from that study suggested that except in religious homes even when there were sufficient complements of staff, during certain times of the day, such as meal times, dying residents were left alone. This suggests that the staffing issue alone could not explain this fact.

The quality of nursing and residential home staff has been discussed in Chapter 2 and training will be discussed in Chapter 8. Suffice it to say, that OU Study (1) revealed great variation in the quality of staff between homes, something that was reflected in their remuneration. Care assistants were generally unqualified, ranging in age from 16 years to near retirement, and expected to undertake work which ranged from nursing care to cooking and cleaning. Quite a number of staff interviewed in both OU Studies had two part time jobs in the home, one as a senior carer and another as a cook or cleaner.

Conclusion

Death in homes has been described as physically uncomfortable with residents suffering from pain, respiratory problems, and emotional distress (OU Study (1); Forbes 2001). Staff often lack the skills to address these and rarely involve outside professionals to help with areas of difficulty (ibid.).

In addition caring for dying residents has resource implications for homes as well as for external providers of health care (see Chapter 7). Home staffing issues have been referred to in this chapter, but clearly the additional burden placed on carers when one resident requires 'intensive caring' has implications for not only the care of other residents and their relatives but also the physical and emotional resources of the staff. Regardless of the burden that staff experience, caring for their residents is seen as their primary obligation and when a resident is terminally ill this is their last opportunity to do it well. The next chapter explores the impact on a home when a resident dies.

References

Ackermann, R.J. (2001) Nursing home practice. Strategies to manage most acute and chronic illnesses without hospitalization. *Geriatrics*, **56**(5), 37, 40, 43–4 passim.

Ackermann, R.J. and Kemle, K.A. (1999) Death in a nursing home with active medical management. *Annals of Long-Term Care*, **7**(8), 313–19.

Baer, W.M. and Hanson, L.C. (2000) Families' perception of the added value of hospice in the nursing home. *Journal of the American Geriatrics Society*, **48**, 879–82.

Berger, A. (2001) Palliative care in long-term-care facilities — a comprehensive model. *Journal of the American Geriatrics Society*, **49**(11), 1570–1.

Casarett, D.J., Hirshman, K.B., and Henry, M.R. (2001) Does hospice have a role in nursing home care at the end of life? *Journal of the American Geriatrics Society*, **49**, 1493–8.

Engle, V.F., Graney, M.J., and Chan, A. (2001) Accuracy and bias of licensed practical nurse and nursing assistant ratings of nursing home residents' pain. *Journal of Gerontology*, **56**A(7), M405–M411.

Fisher, S.E., Burgio, L.D., Thorn, B.E., Allen-Burge, R., Gerstle, J., Roth, D.L., and Allen, S.J. (2002) Pain assessment and management in cognitively impaired nursing home residents: Association of certified nursing assistant pain report, minimum data set pain report, and analgesic medication use. *Journal of the American Geriatrics Society*, **50**, 152–6.

Flacker, J.M., Won, A., Kiely, D.K., and Hoputaife, I. (2001) Different perceptions of end-of-life care in long-term care. *Journal of Palliative Medicine*, **4**(1), 9–13.

Forbes, S. (2001) This is heaven's waiting room: End of life in one nursing home. *Journal of Gerontological Nursing*, November, 37–45.

Froggatt, K. (2000) *Palliative Care Education in Nursing Homes*. Abridged Report of an Evaluation for Macmillan Cancer Relief. Macmillan Cancer Relief, London.

Froggatt, K.A. (2001) Palliative care and nursing homes: Where next? *Palliative Medicine*, **15**, 42–8.

Gagliese, L. and Melzack, R. (1997) Chronic pain in elderly people. *Pain*, **70**, 3–14.

Hall, P., Schroder, C., and Weaver, L. (2002) The last 48 hours of life in long-term care: A focussed chart audit. *Journal of the American Geriatrics Society*, **50**(3), 501–6.

Hanson, L.C. and Henderson, M. (2000) Care of the dying in long-term care settings. *Clinics in Geriatric Medicine*, **16**(2), 225–37.

Hanson, L.C., Henderson, M., and Menon, M. (2002) As individual as death itself: A focus group study of terminal care in nursing homes. *Journal of Palliative Medicine*, **5**(1), 117–25.

Helme, R.D. and Gibson, S.J. (2001) The epidemiology of pain in elderly people. *Clinics in Geriatrics Medicine*, **17**(3), 417.

Hockey, J. (1990) *Experiences of Death*. Edinburgh University Press, Edinburgh.

Howarth, G. (1998) 'Just live for today': Living, caring, ageing, and dying. *Ageing and Society*, **18**, 673–89.

Katz, J.T., Komaromy, C., and Sidell, M. (1999) Understanding palliative care in residential and nursing homes. *International Journal of Palliative Nursing*, **5**(2), 58–64.

Komaromy, C., Sidell, M., and Katz, J.T. (2000) The quality of terminal care in residential and nursing homes. *International Journal of Palliative Nursing* , **6**(4), 192–204.

Miller, S.C., Mor, V., Wu, N., Gozalo, P., and Lapane, K. (2002) Does receipt of hospice care in nursing homes improve the management of pain at the end of life? *Journal of the American Geriatrics Society*, **50**, 507–15.

Maddocks, I. and Parker, D. (2001) Palliative care in nursing homes, in J. Addington-Hall and I. Higginson (eds) *Palliative Care for Non-Cancer Patients*. Oxford University Press, Oxford, 147–57.

Moss, M. and Moss, S. (1996) The impact of family deaths on older people. *Bereavement Care*, **15**(3), 26–27.

Peace, S.M., Kellaher, L. and Willcocks, D.M. (1997) *Re-evaluating residential care*. Open University Press, Buckingham.

Travis, S.S., Loving, G., McClanahan, F.l., and Bernard, M. (2001) Hospitalization patterns and palliation in the last year of life among residents in long-term care. *The Gerontologist*, **41**(2), 153–60.

Walsh, K., King, M., Jones, L., Tookman, A., and Blizard, R. (2002) Spiritual beliefs may affect outcome of bereavement: Prospective study. *British Medical Journal*, **324**(7353).

Chapter 5

Dealing with death

Jeanne Katz

Introduction

Chapter 3 has indicated that care staff frequently encounter residents' deaths, either in the home or shortly after admission to hospital and that this clearly has an impact on staff morale. Chapter 4 demonstrated some of the difficulties carers face in dealing with dying residents, and focused particularly on the challenges of assessing and addressing the needs of dying residents. This chapter considers how carers manage the deaths of residents and the impact death has on home staff. Much of the data presented come from the OU Study (1) as there is a dearth of research information about this topic. Chapter 6 will explore the ways in which staff care for other residents and relatives following a death.

As noted in Chapter 2, the introduction of the National Minimum Standards for Care Homes in 2002 includes a standard for registered managers specifying that significant life events are managed effectively. Hitherto there was little direction to managers in relation to managing death in these settings either in relation to the practical issues involved or with regard to the impact on staff morale. The exception to this was *A Better Home Life* (CPA 1996) which specified in detail policies and procedures in relation to issues around dying and death.

A Better Home Life (CPA 1996) was published whilst OU Study (1) was underway but it was clear from the findings that few of its suggested strategies nor the more limited suggestions from the earlier code of practice *Home Life* had yet percolated through to the homes. The OU Study (1) provided the first substantive data about 'normal practice' for care homes in dealing with death. The survey asked home managers to supply any written documentation in relation to managing death in the homes; in the detailed interviews, home managers were asked to describe their normal procedures following a resident's death. Many of these practices were 'verified' by the researchers during the case study periods.

In 1995 just under half of the homes surveyed (200 of 412) had written policies regarding how to handle a death and all the Local Authority homes demonstrated particularly good practice. Having these displayed in the home's office meant ready access to this information. These policies usually included instructions about notifying the officer in charge of the home, if the body was found by another resident or a carer; notifying the GP and asking for the body to be certified as dead; informing the family, and calling the funeral director.

Procedures when a resident dies

Irrespective of whether they followed a specific policy in relation to caring for deceased residents or not, care homes in OU Study (1) responded in similar ways when a resident died in their own room or away from other residents. Many of the variations to the practices detailed below related to the physical layout of the home and access for undertakers to different areas of the home.

The carer discovering the body usually summoned the most senior person on duty to observe the 'deceased' resident. Even where there were no trained nurses on duty (such as in residential homes) managers noted that before calling the GP they looked for vital signs of life.

> You're obviously looking for pulse, pupil reaction, skin tone. Peoples' features change, that sounds strange but we've seen it when they die. They either go a lot more relaxed or they go very pointed and you can tell, there's a marked change in their features and that's one of the things that always seems to make us think... As I say, pulse, warmth, pupil reaction...

Following agreement that the resident had died, the next step was usually to segregate the body if possible, close the door to the room and take steps to ensure that other residents would not attempt to see the deceased. In most cases, the body was left in the room where the person had died (usually the bedroom) with minimal intervention—straightening the limbs and tidying the hair. It was important for home staff to feel that the body was in a fit condition for relatives to view.

At this point the most senior person on duty would return to the office, phone the GP practice and request that a GP certify the death, notify the relatives, and also check the disposal arrangements before calling the funeral director. A number of administrative procedures also needed to be carried out in relation to the financing of the resident and settling of fees. The resident's personal possessions needed to be itemized and kept in the safe for the relatives to collect.

Lack of clarity about resident's wishes for disposal is one of the greatest obstacles to unproblematic handling of a death. (This also applies to advance directives which is much more common in the United States than currently in the United Kingdom.) *A Better Home Life* (CPA 1996) noted the difficulties in facilitating residents to talk about these and other related issues, and pointed out the sensitivity and compassion required to elicit this information which may emerge at an 'inconvenient' time for carers. Indeed *A Better Home Life* included a list of information necessary for homes to deal with deceased residents.

As with hospital patients, information about disposal wishes is rarely gathered from residents in care homes despite the relevant question on the admission form. Similar to findings in Froggatt's case study of four nursing homes (2000), in OU Study (1) some older people were asked this question on admission to the home. However in most care homes if this was found out, it happened during an assessment or in casual discussion after the resident had been in the home for some months once carers felt that they had developed a close enough relationship with residents to ask such sensitive questions. Disposal preferences were essential information in order to know which type of death certificate (for burial or cremation) the GP was required to complete after death. A Local Authority home used the following procedure:

> The disposal details are actually a part of the case history, burial/cremation and who the undertakers are and the next of kin, the person who is to be contacted. So that is down already. It is not general practice to ask people how they want to be dealt with immediately, that does not seem to be something that people can talk about. People have great difficulty in talking about death and dying and tend not to want to address it.

GPs carried out death certification in various ways. This depended primarily on their familiarity with the resident and their assessment of the home staff. A minority of all types of homes reported that GPs did not necessarily come in to certify the death. Sometimes they came immediately, in other cases GPs relied on the experience of staff, even in residential homes, to recognize death. In some nursing homes, nurses were permitted to certify the death as the following quote demonstrates:

> Our staff are trained. First level nurses are covered to certify patients during the night, so that if we know that a patient is likely to die, the GP is asked to write in the patient's case notes that they are satisfied with the nursing staff to certify.

When GPs visited to certify a death, the contact with the deceased was often brief, more time being spent with care staff or relatives if they were present. In the case of an expected death the GP would sometimes arrange to go to the local undertaker and certify the body there. This is not good practice as it places a responsibility on the home staff for which they are not legally covered. Additionally family members may want to see a death certificate or even meet with the general practitioner when s/he comes to certify death, and therefore signing the death certificate at the undertaker's prevents the family from meeting the GP.

Laying out the body or last offices

Several homes had policies not to interfere with the body whilst it was still warm:

> I teach the young staff to sit with the body because it shows respect and you don't want to start laying out a person while they are still warm; you have to be respect-ful don't you and I think its very important to relatives.

In OU Study (1) most homes, other than those with a religious affiliation, had abandoned the procedure of laying out. Two justifications were provided for this—one related to the fact that this is part of the funeral directors' role and the other was that it was an antiquated practice associated with hospitals. However homes affiliated with a religious order still carried out 'last offices'— these were mostly homes from the voluntary sector. This practice entails washing the body, straightening the limbs, plugging the orifices, and securing the jaw:

> We tend to straighten them out immediately. The first thing we do is (we tend to have them on their side or propped up with pillows for comfort) and so we lie them flat. We generally leave it for about half an hour because that's as long as it takes you to do phone calls and let people know and then we go in and wash them down and do formally all the last offices and then the arrangements get taken over by their family.

Some non-denominational homes also called the priest if they had instruc-tions from the deceased. And then they proceeded to care for the body.

> After that we went back and washed Eileen's body and she used to wear a wig and I used to wash and dress the wig. We washed her and talked to her as 'I am just going to turn you over Eileen and do your back and put a clean nightie on', made sure her teeth were in, and put her wig on made her look nice, a little cushion just under the chin, the covers up over the cushion but not over the face and she looked so peaceful, she really looked so much younger, yes, it really was lovely. . . I have always been taught that you might think that they don't know anything but I believe that they still hear. I just feel that they can still hear, I don't know whether I am right or wrong but that is the way we treat them, you know, talk to them not over them or about them.

Generally staff wanted the deceased to look as clean, comfortable, and 'natural' as possible particularly in case relatives should want to see the deceased after death. Staff members were often disappointed when relatives did not visit.

Only a few homes had experience of handling the death of a resident from an ethnic minority. Local Authority homes were more likely to be aware of different cultural and religious practices and had these incorporated in their 'procedures':

> We have to follow certain procedures and we have information on people who die that belong to different religions. The ones who can't be touched obviously and those kinds. We have that in the code of practice, and we do refer back to it occasionally, just to remind ourselves that this could happen and so far it hasn't; we haven't been asked to care for anyone from one of the ethnic minorities, but that shouldn't stop us from being aware that there are different practices for people from other religions.

Differences other than religious were not acknowledged by homes in the OU Study (1). This could be explained by the fact that most of the residents were homogeneous (white British born) and that the study took place only in England and did not include the other countries of the United Kingdom. There were no reported deaths from AIDS and no respondents talked about same sex relationships and implications thereof.

Deceased residents were usually left in their own bed, as 'lifelike' as possible. Viewing the body was rarely offered as an option to residents, but if asked managers did not refuse access:

> Those who wanted to had already been in to see her. The majority of them no, they would rather stay out of the way.

The length of time a body of a deceased resident remained in the homes varied. The funeral director was called as soon as death was certified and disposal arrangements had been clarified. Usually funeral directors came to remove the body about an hour after the death. Managers sometimes called the funeral directors later if relatives wanted to come to the home and sit with the body. The following account from a Local Authority home manager was very unusual but illustrates good practice from a number of points of view, not least that the death was not hidden from fellow residents:

> She died in the morning and we left her in that chair until 6 o'clock in the evening. The doctor had certified but we left her in the chair until the family said it was alright for her to go, and the family spent all day. It was early morning when she died. They spent the whole of the day coming in and mourning and doing whatever they needed to do the ritual in the way that was right for them. And all we did was check that everybody was alright and that they had food and drink all day. And we felt that it was important and I think the family felt that was best for them as well. They were very happy with that and it is no problem at all. There is no

problem at all, there is no problem about leaving people here. It is not a secret that somebody has died.

Homes affiliated to a religious order sometimes have their own chapel of rest where the body could stay if the family wished. In some homes the body was often returned to the chapel the night before the funeral service and a vigil took place:

> We have a chapel and so it is not just die and disappearing you know. We lay them out and the undertaker takes them away. They come back in, we have a service here for them very often.

Dying in a public area is particularly difficult for staff to manage. The usual procedure in these cases is that staff attempt to manoeuvre the body into a private space or alternatively, they prevent residents from using this area till the body has been taken away. Unexpected deaths in public places of residents who had not seen their GP during the previous fortnight, create particular difficulties for staff as the body has to remain *in situ* till the police arrive or coroner gives permission to move the body. Under these circumstances staff found it hard to maintain the equilibrium in the home.

Removing the body

Findings from OU Study (1) revealed that despite home managers' preferences for being open about death and statements that they disapproved of bodies going out the back door, regardless of the category of home, removing the body was concealed from other residents. It was generally believed that residents should be protected from deaths of co-residents and bodies should be removed as discreetly as possible. Doors were closed or curtains drawn or residents were shepherded away from the public areas to their rooms. In most instances the body was removed from the bedroom via the nearest exit. Exceptions to this occurred if there were practical difficulties or if it meant taking the body through the reception area of the home at a time when residents were present.

> We try to arrange to do it at a time when there aren't many residents around. I think it can be a little bit distressing for them.

Residents were often prevented from observing what was happening:

> They take the body out in a body bag and leave the trolley at the bottom of the steps. The residents don't know because all the doors are shut and somebody is on guard while it's happening.

A number of managers found the manner in which bodies were removed very distressing and upsetting and sought to protect residents from the sight and the concept that the same would happen to them. This has been corroborated in other settings where residents have noted that the same trolley is used for all dead bodies and find the sight appalling.

> I won't say to residents, 'Go away, a coffin's coming past' or 'a body's coming past.' But neither will I invite them to be there because I think it matters to them to know that they will be going out in a dignified way and a golf bag is not.

Sometimes the removal of bodies was particularly difficult:

> They put them into the lift and literally stand the body on the trolley and bring it down. It is not a very nice experience, you have got to think of it as a shell then. Say it was three o'clock in the afternoon we draw the curtains in the lounge and inform the day centre so they keep their residents [away], because its not a nice thing to see, we try and use the back exit door there.

Most managers found the sight of their residents standing up in body bags in tiny lifts extremely distressing and undignified. They expressed relief when bodies could be removed at night with minimal disruption to home life and other residents. In most accounts, funeral directors were very co-operative and homes had well established links with local firms.

Once the body was removed, the room was cleared of the deceased resident's possessions and prepared for the next occupant.

Supporting staff after a bereavement

Following a resident's death, managers strive to maintain normal routines in order to maintain an equilibrium for surviving residents who are seen to react badly to changes in staff demeanour. Managers have a difficult task to balance carers' needs for practical and emotional support and at the same time ensure that other residents are appropriately cared for. Their ability to do this depends both on resource and training issues, but also the home's ethos in relation to acknowledging individual carers' strengths and frailties plays an important role.

Practical support

A dying or deceased resident creates workload implications for the home. Staffing levels rarely take into account the additional work that a death creates. The manager withdraws into the office to make phone calls and then may spend time talking to relatives or GPs and possibly helping the funeral directors remove the body. More time is taken up breaking the news to other carers and all the residents. Some funerals are planned from the home and this too creates additional work.

Emotional support

There is little dispute that staff working in care homes require emotional support when a resident is dying or has died (Working Party on Clinical Guidelines in Palliative Care 1997; OU Study (1)). As noted in the previous chapter, the intensity of the relationships that carers have with residents resembles that of families and therefore they may require bereavement support in the same way as family members (Hanson and Henderson 2000). Managers in the OU Study (1) observed that carers became particularly attached to some residents and often became distressed as death neared. Many carers are young with little personal experience of dealing with dying and death. In some homes key workers are appointed for residents, and their emotional involvement can be intensive.

For managers the challenge is therefore how to ensure that carers are able to carry on with their work as well as acknowledging their grief (Katz *et al.* 2000, 2001). Several factors influence whether this is accomplished satisfactorily (Katz 2002). The first concerns how staff are informed about a death; the second relates to how their bereavement needs are addressed; and the third explores their options for concluding their work with the deceased, by bidding them farewell.

Informing staff about a death

In OU Study (1), managers said that their policy was not to inform off-duty colleagues that a resident had died. They justified this practice by suggesting that it took up valuable staff time to call off-duty colleagues, phone calls were expensive and that it was unprofessional to disturb carers' off-duty time. Yet despite management policies, carers who were on duty when the death occurred often phoned their colleagues at home and this triggered the snowballing of the information. Whilst acknowledging the virtue of the policy deemed to protect their private lives, many carers suggested that they wanted to know when off-duty if a resident to whom they were particularly attached had died.

There were certain exceptions to the rule of not informing off-duty staff. These included where staff had specifically requested notification or were identified by the manager as particularly vulnerable or were seen to be especially close to the dying person or relatives:

> The key worker was actually off sick so we phoned her at home to tell her because she would want to know. We don't like them to just come in and find out; we either try to get in touch with them, either ring them or pop round. It really does depend on how close they are to that resident. If they are just generally looking after them, you know, not a key worker or co-worker then they will be told when they come on this shift that X passed away at this time.

A few homes acknowledged that other visitors to the homes should also be advised:

> The hairdresser cries just like the rest of us—she is included, she is always told before she comes to work, because she does take a great interest in them and so does the chiropodist, she has been here a long time as well.

However, the reality is that most care staff discover that a resident has died when they next report for duty. They find out in various unplanned ways, these include meeting another staff member at the front door, looking in the diary, case notes or on the notice board, at a staff meeting, finding the resident missing, or the worst case scenario—someone else in the bed. One manager tried to plan ways in which the next shift would be informed:

> If it happens at night and you have a morning shift coming on then you station someone at the door and tell them as they come on duty. It doesn't always work. Sometimes for some reason you'll miss someone, you tend to catch them before they are about to come on shift and again depending on how upset they are, you leave them in the staff room. You have to deal with them as you would an upset relative, help them through it. Usually they will get over it and continue the shift but if they weren't [able to continue] then we would obviously take them home.

Ensuring that staff members who have been on holiday or away from the home for some time are appropriately informed is important. In the same way as information about preferences are extracted from residents, carers could be enabled to choose how they would like to receive this information. This would reduce the possibility that carers are so distressed by the news that they find it hard to function.

Legitimating carers' grief

In many care homes residents have little contact with their remaining families and friends—they live far away, may be emotionally distant, or dislike the care environment (Hanson and Henderson 2000). Care staff often assume the role of in loco family members and take deaths of residents very personally (Forbes 2001). This section explores ways in which managers strive to acknowledge the relationships between carers and residents and the implications for the former when the latter die.

In OU Study (1) about half the managers viewed supporting their staff as an integral part of their job. However they felt they were hampered on two counts from providing this support successfully. First they lacked the required counselling skills to do this well and second they lacked time. Staffing levels meant that they were rarely freed to spend sufficient time supporting carers after a death (because they were sorting out practical issues in relation to the deceased) nor could they allocate another senior member of staff to this task.

The study suggested that the bereavement needs of carers could be separated into several components. First, carers need reassurance that they have done all that they could to make the deceased comfortable and secure. This reassurance could emerge from rehearsing the events that surrounded the death, something counselling texts emphasize as important (e.g. Davy and Ellis 2000). Questions that need answering for those both present at the death and those who were absent, relate to the cause and circumstances of the death. Carers not on the premises at the time will want to know whether the death was painless and peaceful, was the resident alone, and what part, if any, did the relatives play? These concerns mirror those of surviving residents (OU Study (1)).

Second, carers need permission to repress or express their feelings, whichever works for them. In OU Study (1), carers coped with their emotions in a variety of ways, one of which was sharing their feelings with one another:

> Actually they have been very fond of who ever it is that's died and they do grieve, they do weep. . . They talk to each other and we talk to them and let them express their grief and they can have a little memento of the person if they want, a photograph.

As in other settings (Katz 1996) senior staff role-modelled to junior carers what they believed to be acceptable demonstration of emotions. In some homes care staff were discouraged from crying in front of relatives but in most homes this was acceptable as long as carers were able to return to their duties. Most carers noted that once they had had an opportunity to talk about the life and death of the deceased resident with colleagues and with relatives (if appropriate) they had to get on with the job. This was more difficult when there was a 'run' of deaths, which not only drained staff emotionally but also placed a lot of pressure on carrying out practical tasks. This was particularly taxing for managers who were not only coping with the emotional and practical demands of junior staff, relatives, and support staff, but also with their own grief and often exhaustion.

Bidding farewell to deceased residents and their relatives

Carers need to feel that they have closure with deceased residents and their relatives. For some this means viewing the body in the home but this is often not practical as carers may be off duty or relatives may be present. Carers find the transitional relationships with relatives very difficult and often are lost for words when relatives come in to the home after the death. Both the OU Studies indicated that providing training in communication skills and bereavement care may increase carers' confidence as well as competence in areas such as these.

Attending funerals is for many carers their last opportunity to do something for the resident and a way of communicating positively with relatives. *A Better Home Life* (CPA 1996) recommended that the staff should be transported to funerals and their rosters adjusted so that they could attend. But, attending funerals is sometimes not practical because of the timing or location of the funeral as well as staffing issues (OU Study (1)). Nevertheless unless the funeral took place far from the home, in which case a wreath was sent, home staff were represented at residents' funerals. Almost half the home managers saw attending funerals as part of their job. The remaining managers asked the staff team to decide who should attend the funeral. At some funerals there were no mourners other than care staff. Although staff usually attended in work time, care staff often attend funerals when off duty despite the fact that they were rarely compensated:

> Some staff go in their own time, it's their choice if they want to. (For the last funeral) both of us went and took some residents with us and a lot of the staff that were off-duty went anyway. Some can't go because they are at work. . . We had a gentleman who died and he had no family at all and we had him taken over to the little chapel and then up to the crem and you couldn't have wished for a nicer funeral you know. All the residents went and all the staff because he had nobody he thought of us as his family, even the district nurses went, then they all came back here and we felt as if we did our part and had nothing to regret.

Conclusion

Dealing with death in care homes poses a number of challenges for staff. The practical implications are time consuming and the whole experience can be emotionally draining. The next chapter will explore the ways in which homes care for other residents and relatives when a resident is dying or has died. As Chapters 8 and 9 will demonstrate, increasing managers' and carers' knowledge about different aspects of palliative and bereavement care may directly impact on the ways in which they manage death in care homes.

References

Centre for Policy on Ageing (1996) *A Better Home Life*. Centre for Policy on Ageing, London.

Davy, J. and Ellis, S. (2000) *Counselling Skills in Palliative Care*. Open University Press, Buckingham.

Forbes, S. (2001) This is heaven's waiting room: End of life in one nursing home. *Journal of Gerontological Nursing*, November, 37–45.

Froggatt, K. (2000) *Palliative Care Education in Nursing Homes*. Abridged Report of an Evaluation for Macmillan Cancer Relief, Macmillan Cancer Relief.

Froggatt, K.A. (2001) Palliative care and nursing homes: Where next? *Palliative Medicine*, **15**, 42–8.

Hanson, L.C. and Henderson, M. (2000) Care of the dying in long-term care settings. *Clinics in Geriatric Medicine*, **16**(2), 225–37.

Hanson, L.C., Henderson, M., and Menon, M. (2002) As individual as death itself: A focus group study of terminal care in nursing homes, *Journal of Palliative Medicine*, **5**(1), 117–25.

Katz, J. (1996) Nurses' perceptions of stress when working with dying patients on a cancer ward in Howarth, G. and Jupp, P.C. (eds.), *Contemporary Issues in the Sociology of Death, Dying and Disposal*. Macmillan, London, 124–136.

Katz, J.T., Komaromy, C., and Sidell, M. (2000) Death in homes: Bereavement needs of residents, relatives and staff. *International Journal of Palliative Nursing*, **6**(6), 274–79.

Katz, J.S., Sidell, M., and Komaromy, C. (2001) Dying in long term care facilities: Support needs of other residents, relatives and staff. *American Journal of Hospice & Palliative Care*, September/October, **18**(5), 321–26.

Katz, J.S. (2002) Managing loss in care homes, in J. Reynolds, J. Henderson, J. Seden, J. Charlesworth, and A. Bullman (eds) *The Managing Care Reader*. Routledge, London.

Working Party on Clinical Guidelines in Palliative Care (1997) *Changing Gear: Guidelines for Managing the Last Days of Life in Adults*. National Council for Hospice and Specialist Palliative Care Services, London.

Chapter 6

The needs of relatives and other residents when a death occurs

Carol Komaromy

The status of death in care homes

One of the most demanding aspects of the role of care staff in homes for older people is that of having to manage the difficult boundary between life and death. Care staff need to be able to care for living and dying residents in the same setting and even simultaneously on the same shifts. They also have to cope with any grief reactions of all those concerned, including their own, following the death of home residents. It is clear from this that, for care staff, being able to meet the needs of relatives and other residents following a resident's death in a care home is beset with inherent tensions and managing these adds a further level of complexity to their already demanding care role. This chapter draws on ethnographic data from OU Study (1) (Sidell *et al.* 1997) to consider some of the difficulties that are faced by care home staff in meeting the needs of relatives and residents following death. The data are drawn from 12 case studies and include observations at and around the time of death, interviews with residents, relatives of deceased residents, and care home staff.

Death at the end of a long life has been constructed in Western society as 'natural and timely' (Komaromy and Hockey 2001). But staff in care homes for older people are also concerned to use the event of death as a way of returning meaning to a life in which meaning might have been lost, and so death is also constructed as a significant event (Komaromy 2000). Part of this construction is played out in death-bed scenes in what Goffman would call 'dramaturgical events' (Goffman 1959).

Howarth (1996) in her study of funeral directors uses the ideas of Goffman to explain their performance on the 'stage' of death. Most of this is front stage where the public viewing of bodies takes place and what happens back stage is part of the preparation for this performance. Here the impression of a peaceful death inscribed upon the body of the corpse was what was being produced. Likewise, in care homes, the staff needed to present a coherent impression of sad and significant death as a natural and timely event at the end of a long life. This was conveyed through their demeanour around the time of death. But death can only be produced in this way if the actors involved are aware of what is taking place and therefore some degree of preparation for death is essential. Not surprisingly, all of this is thrown into chaos at the time of sudden death and, when this happens, staff and family seek out devices to compensate for both their lack of expectation of and their absence at the time of death. Accounts from OU Study (1) confirm that sudden death creates enormous distress and is something that most staff dread, even though it is not a regular occurrence, accounting as it did for only 10 per cent of all deaths (Sidell *et al.* 1997). As with all other forms of care, the registered managers are ultimately responsible for the way in which death in homes is managed and a key aspect of their orchestration of death includes the way in which information is conveyed to family and other residents. Chapter 3 described how the period of dying was narrowly confined to the last few weeks or even days of life. Home care staff preferred the bedside vigil to be held by a family member of the dying resident, but as discussed later, this did not necessarily apply to those deaths that were likely to occur at night.

It was clear from listening to accounts given by both the relatives of deceased residents and also surviving residents that, in most homes, the provision of information around the time of death to relatives took precedence over that given to other residents, regardless of the quality of these relationships. However, there were striking differences between many of the homes in terms of how the disclosure of information was handled. For example, some homes had written policies which laid down the practices that should be adhered to at the time of and immediately following death. In other homes the registered managers took sole charge of who was told what and when. There were also homes in which the practices were less clear, so that some staff expressed feelings of insecurity about what it was permissible to say to family and other residents. Terms like 'very poorly' which Froggatt (2001) describes in her nursing home study were used as safer euphemistic alternatives, so that residents were not allocated a dying status. But in most homes the relationship between the home staff, most particularly the registered manager, and the family and friends of dying or deceased residents was pivotal to the way in which bad news about a death was broken.

It is not surprising that when registered managers had a good relationship with visiting family and friends they felt more able to support them through the difficult period of a resident's terminal illness. This was often because they had established a level of familiarity which made support easier to give at such times of vulnerability. In homes in which there was a long-standing and close relationship with a close family member the head of home might visit them to break the news and to be with them, if they knew that they were alone. Conversely, registered managers and care staff found it very difficult to cope with relatives who did not appear to be interested in a particular resident. If family and friends had previously been infrequent visitors to the home, care staff experienced difficulty in establishing rapport when residents were thought to be dying. Carers and heads of homes had several explanations for these infrequent visits, which ranged from the family's lack of caring to their guilt because they had 'put' the resident in a home. The registered manager of a private residential home told us:

> I'm afraid she didn't get very good back up from her family. She had three children who didn't come very often. She used to get very upset about it, which was understandable — they only had one mother.

Staff also expressed resentment about the contrast between 'a good turn out' at a resident's funeral and the lack of visitors during their stay in the home.

Breaking the news of death to family and friends

Whether formally recognized or established over time through practice and routine, breaking the news of a death was usually part of the role of the registered home manager. The care staff maintained that informing relatives of the death of a resident was something that they disliked doing and were pleased that the head of home usually undertook this task. Many care staff thought that this is what the senior staff were paid to do. Indeed in some homes the manager and deputies were on call to deal with deaths and care staff called them out if a death occurred. The senior staff member on duty or the registered home manager/owner would contact the next-of-kin, unless it had been established that they did not want to be told at night.

Despite the expectations and preparation of many of the homes the needs of relatives could be very different from that which home staff anticipated. For example, even though some of the homes provided amenities for overnight accommodation it was unusual for relatives to stay at night, particularly if they lived close to the home and were themselves older people. It was important therefore, that during the terminal phase of a resident's illness, heads of homes made attempts to ascertain what the close family's wishes were about being contacted at night. The son of a resident who died in a private nursing home described the arrangements made to contact him when his mother was close to death:

> Matron, she said, 'We will let you know but not in the middle of the night because there's nothing you can do.' I said, 'Well, no. Thank you. That's a point. No point them ringing me to tell me in the middle of the night Mum had gone.'

This relative's account echoes the sentiments of relatives who did not want to be informed until the next morning. The daughter of a resident who died in a private residential home explained why she did not want to be told in the night:

> She was unconscious and I rang before I went to bed and Janet said, 'Do you want me to ring you? And I said, 'No!' I am on my own and in the middle of the night I would have been too scared to go out, although she said that Gary (partner of home manager and also nephew of the resident) would come for me.

Sometimes when the family were not available the task of breaking the news could be even more difficult. When a resident in Eden Lodge called John was dying, his nephew was aware that his uncle was very ill but not that he was dying and had decided to continue with his holiday plans. When John's nephew telephoned the home from his holiday resort abroad he was told that his uncle's condition was relatively stable. John died just 20 minutes later and the person in charge of that unit then had to contact John's nephew to tell him the bad news. Not only did he describe this as extremely difficult, but also he located part of the distress in the embarrassment that this caused him. There were clearly practical reasons for John's nephew to know when his uncle might die but it would be reasonable to speculate that, in general, home staff are invested with an expectation of an ability to predict the time of death.

The funeral and the removal of belongings

Wherever possible registered managers elicited the wishes for disposal before the death occurred. But, as noted in the previous chapters, frequently the subject of disposal was not discussed and there were many occasions when staff had to find out the family's wishes after the death as well as being on hand to give guidance and advice.

The experience of relatives at the time of a death will vary depending on the level of attachment to the resident and it is a time of mixed emotions and practicalities concerning official formalities, possessions, and funerals. From the findings of OU Study (1), following a resident's death the focus was largely upon the practical arrangements and involved frequent negotiations over who would perform what tasks. Part of the support which staff gave to friends and relatives after a resident's death was advice about the required formal procedures surrounding the registration of death and funeral arrangements. Several heads of homes commented that it was difficult for the family to collect the death certificate from the GP and many of them arranged for the certificate to be collected from the home instead.

In all settings in which death occurs relatives and friends raised concerns about the way in which the removal of belongings was managed. Family was invited to collect belongings of deceased residents. The length of time in which they could collect them from the resident's former room largely depended upon occupancy levels and some homes needed to empty the room within two days of the death. If the family were unable to collect any belongings these were usually kept in a storeroom in the home. In some homes, registered managers explained that they needed to empty the room within a week of the resident's death. The sister of a resident described how together with her nieces she had to remove her brother's belongings a few days after the death:

> I went up there to meet his daughters a couple of days afterwards because they wanted the room for someone else and they wanted all the things cleared out.

The issue of collecting belongings after death also emphasizes that homes are also businesses and the demands of full-occupancy conflicted with the need to maintain the significant and sensitive nature of death. Other homes left the room untouched until the family came to collect belongings. However this was managed, returning to the home was difficult for many relatives as the following quote from a relative of a resident who died in a private residential home illustrates:

> We went quite soon after mum died and got that job done. We thought it was best to get it done and out of the way. I want to go to see the residents but not yet. I can't go yet, it's too hard!

After the funeral a few homes contacted the family and invited them to special events in the home. Sometimes a relative or friend would continue to visit other residents with whom they had established a relationship. The daughter of a resident who died in a rural home told us:

> Oh yes! I've been back. I mean, we used to go in there and sit in there and talk to them (two of the other residents) as much as we did to mum!

Homes in small, contained rural communities were more likely to stay in touch with the family because care staff could maintain informal local contact, through fund-raising or visiting relatives who had been left with no family. For example, one home employed the daughter of a deceased resident as an activities officer at a time when she was coping with the deaths of both parents and her son's severe psychotic breakdown.

The practice in these homes appears to be the exception and most of the registered managers observed that the family did not return after the resident's death. Some relatives commented that although they wanted to return to the home and had promised to do so, they found it much too painful to return.

As time progressed it seemed that this became more difficult. The overwhelming number of friends and relatives did not return and no contact was made by either party.

Notifying other residents about a death in the home

At the time of dying and death relatives and friends of deceased residents were more likely to be informed and supported than other residents in the home, regardless of the relationship between residents. Only when any relatives had been informed of a death, did the staff turn their attention to the other residents. This was the case even in homes in which there was an openness about death and dying, such as Catholic homes. Here although the end of life was seen as an important preparation for death, relatives' needs took precedence over those of fellow residents. The news of a death needed to be given in a way which took into account the perceived needs of other residents, which included an assumed concern about their own demise. For example, many registered managers, like this head of a voluntary home, commented that residents wanted to know whether the person had died peacefully, painlessly, and whether they were alone:

> When we have had a death residents will discuss it amongst themselves and they will always ask you what has happened and how were they and things like that. One of the biggest questions that we are asked by a lot by relatives and residents is 'were they alone?' I think that is one of everybody's fears isn't it that you die on your own.

In most of the homes in OU Study (1) some of the residents, but by no means all, were told when someone died. As with most other information, the registered manager judged what to say to surviving residents both before and after a resident's death. His or her judgement was likely to be based upon two key aspects. First, the perceived closeness of the relationship between the surviving resident and the deceased person and second, the ability of the surviving resident to comprehend the news.

Closeness in terms of relationships is a key concern but many of the larger homes were spatially divided. In many care homes residents were segregated from one another into smaller units in an attempt to reduce an institutionalized environment and produce a sense of homeliness. The division of residents was usually made according to their care needs and/or the size of the home population. In large homes that were divided into units the residents might only meet up for special occasions like Christmas. Other homes had less rigid boundaries, but still segregated residents into different lounge and dining areas. Therefore, in homes with over twenty residents it was unlikely that they would all know each other. Eden Lodge was a group-living home where the residents fell into three broad categories: those who were ambulant, those who were immobile, and those who were categorized as 'elderly mentally infirm' (EMI). The following account taken from field notes describes what happened when John died in Eden Lodge:

> When staff arrived on duty the following day they were greeted with the news of John's death. They expressed both sadness and relief. None of the staff in the home was particularly upset and the care assistant who had found John's body was off duty. In the EMI unit the staff drank their coffee at the same time as feeding the residents their breakfast. They talked to each other about having told the residents in the other units about John's death. It seemed that they assumed that none of the residents around them was capable of absorbing the information and felt comfortable talking to one another about their feelings in the presence of residents. The conversation began to focus on a discussion of personal loss and how the staff manage their own losses alongside the deaths of residents with a very poor quality of life. The staff also talked about how they got close to some of the residents and how while they knew that this was 'wrong' they couldn't help becoming attached. One care assistant in the home said: 'We shouldn't get close really but you can't help it.'
>
> The funeral arrangements were to be left to John's nephew who was returning from his holiday. A representative from the home would be sent to the funeral, but no one on duty that day wanted to attend. None of the residents was invited to the funeral because the home staff thought that none of them would want to attend. The staff were pleased that John's nephew would be able to collect the belongings from the room himself because he was coming in the following day.

John's death was striking in the lack of impact it seemed to have on everyone in the home. His death illustrates that knowing other residents personally is not only dependent upon spatial proximity. Those residents who for years had shared the EMI unit with him appeared unaware that he had died and the staff declared that they did not intend telling them. The staff had made it clear that they thought it was inappropriate for him to remain in the home for terminal care and strove to transfer him to hospital. They seemed to have managed an emotional distance through their lack of commitment to the management of his dying and death. Because they viewed John's death as an inappropriate and unwanted event they seemed to remain at an emotional distance from the event. In Goffmanesque terms this performance did not need to convey the sanctioned peaceful, meaningful, and sad death. The staff were not interested in participating in a convincing performance and the surviving residents, as their potential audience, were not acknowledged as being capable of comprehending what was taking place.

But when residents were thought to have formed important relationships the way in which the death of one of them was handled was different. Lily had lived in *Waltham* Nursing Home for 12 years and her death impacted upon those residents who had shared the lounge with her. The following account from field notes describes what happened:

> Lily died at 4 p.m. and Matron was called. She felt for a carotid pulse and delegated two care assistants to straighten Lily's body. A few minutes later Matron intercepted Lily's niece's husband on his way to Lily's room to warn him of the death (he had been notified about Lily's further deterioration). Initially he was reluctant to see Lily but then decided to say good-bye only staying for less than a minute. He was very shocked and upset and said: 'I should have been prepared because I was expecting it, but this is the third death'.
>
> Matron took him to her office and gave him a cup of tea which one of the care assistants was asked to make. Slowly one by one the care assistants on duty came to say good-bye to Lily.
>
> At 5.30 p.m. the GP arrived to certify the death. She held a stethoscope on Lily's chest for three seconds only and pronounced her dead with a nod of the head. The GP then sped out of the room as quickly as she had entered still eating a toffee and talking to Matron about something unrelated to the death. Lily was not mentioned.
>
> Matron then decided to tell the seven residents, whom she believed would want to know that Lily had died. She did so individually using these words:
>
> I'm very sorry to have to tell you that on this day of the Lord at four o'clock Lily passed peacefully away.
>
> Both Winnie and Gladys, two of Lily's friends, immediately became very upset and cried a lot.
>
> Matron decided that she would wash Lily herself and prepare her for the funeral directors. The staff were told to give out the teas while Matron laid Lily out single-handedly. I re-entered the room just as Matron wanted to tidy the room and move the furniture so that the undertakers would have free access via the French doors and so that the removal of the body would remain concealed. She asked me to help her.

There are times in homes when breaking bad news to surviving residents is essential. For example, where married couples lived in a home and shared a room, telling the surviving spouse that their partner was dying or had died could be very difficult. The following account by the registered home manager reveals how one head of home assumed (wrongly) that the partner had understood the condition of his spouse:

> And I said to the girls would you get the wheelchair for me and would you bring Douglas straight down. I sat him by the bed and said, 'Just hold her hand Douglas, I don't think she is very well. I think she is very, very poorly'. And as he sat there she died. He hadn't, he really hadn't a clue, because I had to say to him, 'Douglas I think Edith has died.' And he said, 'What do we do now then, love?' I said, 'Well we are going to leave you with her for a few minutes, so you can say your good-byes in private, then we will come back and sort things out with you.'

Then he said, 'Why, do you think she is going to die?' So he hadn't taken it in that she had died at all!

Another time when residents had to be told that someone had died was when residents shared a room, although the use of shared rooms is diminishing. Sometimes the 'living' resident was moved out of the bedroom into the lounge and registered managers gave accounts of this taking place at night. Registered managers and staff also gave accounts of the roommate not being aware that anything was taking place. However, in one home the staff recounted the effect on a resident whose roommate had died which was that he was unable to sleep with the light off after the death.

One registered manager emphasized that the ways in which residents were told varied. As with most other forms of communication, the disclosure of news to other residents was orchestrated:

> Usually the senior person on duty goes round and tells them individually and if any of them want to speak about it, they've got the opportunity to do so.

Some of the care staff commented that they felt it was inappropriate to break the bad news of a resident's death at night because it might cause distress or disturb their sleep.

Funeral arrangements

Some homes arranged for the funeral cortege to leave from the home and were happy to receive wreaths and flowers after the funeral. Other homes did not feel this was appropriate (see Chapter 9). A small minority of homes, mostly voluntary residential homes which were associated with a religious order, held memorial services on their premises for deceased residents, for the benefit of family, friends, and other residents. A very small number of homes undertook some commemoration of deceased residents, whether through planting a tree or another permanent memorial. Often relatives made donations in the deceased's name and this money was used in a number of ways to improve the services of the home for the surviving residents.

In most homes, although not specifically denied the opportunity, residents rarely attended funerals. Home staff in the case study homes claimed that few residents really wanted to go to funerals and it was unclear whether or not they were specifically invited to do so or whether they had to request to go. The frailer residents had great difficulty in getting around and therefore were less likely to attend funerals than more ambulant ones. In all, relatively few residents attended funerals.

Constraints on staff responding to the needs of relatives, friends, and residents

The constraints on the provision of bereavement care and support to relatives, friends and residents arise at the two levels of awareness and resources. The way in which death is managed and the restriction of the dying period does not allow for an exploration of the needs of relatives and other residents beyond those that coincide with the home's construction of needs. If these needs are measured against a palliative care philosophy and approach in which the dying person and their carers are at the centre of any decision-making process, then it is clear that these needs will be open to different interpretations. But if the management of death and dying were to be orchestrated differently then the heads of home would need to increase their recognition and understanding of the principles and practice of palliative care (see Chapter 9).

This chapter has highlighted how care staff meet the needs of relatives and other residents when a death occurs. It has drawn upon the findings of OU Study 1 to illustrate how registered managers orchestrate the death of a resident as a dual opportunity to confer significance upon death in a way that can bring meaning to that life and construct the death as a sad event. The role of relatives is privileged above that of other residents through the management of information about death, dying, and attendance at the funeral. The emotional impact of a death on relatives, the business needs of the home, and the staff's own needs to separate living from dying residents all constrain those involved in their freedom to express their bereavement needs following the death. Recognizing the dying trajectory as part of a continuum, alongside a palliative care approach that centres on the needs of dying people and their family and friends, would allow for a greater recognition of everyone's needs and help to reduce the burden on staff to tightly manage the boundary between living and dying.

References

Froggatt, K. (2001) Life and death in English nursing homes: Sequestration or transition? *Ageing and Society*, 21. Cambridge University Press, Cambridge, 319–332.

Goffman, E. (1959) *The Presentation of Self in Everyday Life*. Penguin, Harmondworth.

Howarth, G. (1996) *Last Rights: The Work of the Modern Funeral Director*. Baywood Publishing Company, New York.

Komaromy, C. (2000) The sight and sound of death: The management of dead bodies in residential and nursing homes for older people. *Mortality*, 5(3).

Komaromy, C. and Hockey, J. (2001) Naturalising death among older adults in residential care, in J. Hockey, J. Katz, and N. Small (eds) *Grief, Mourning and Death Ritual*. Open University Press, Buckingham, 73–82.

Sidell, M., Katz, J.T., and Komaromy, C. (1997) *Death and Dying in Residential and Nursing Homes for Older People: Examining the case for Palliative Care*, Report to the Department of Health.

Chapter 7

The role of external health workers

Jeanne Katz

Introduction

In the United Kingdom, health care in the community depends first and foremost on the primary health care team, which operates more or less independently of the tertiary hospital sector. This team is made up of a range of health professionals orbiting the general practitioner or family doctor. Members of this team usually include those who work primarily at the surgery premises itself as well as those who work both at the surgery and outside in the community. People dying in the community also receive services from specialist nurses and palliative care teams, the composition, and affiliation of which vary with geographical location. This chapter explores the roles of primary care teams in relation to care homes and also of specialist services available to dying people and makes suggestions in relation to facilitating more seamless care.

The role of the primary health care team is pivotal to caring for people dying outside acute settings. This applies especially to residential and nursing homes where as noted in Chapter 4, care staff may not have the expertise to address all the needs of terminally ill residents. It is important to understand the expectations of both home staff and external health professionals, in particular general practitioners, community nurses, and specialist palliative care nurses in relation to the roles they believe they can play in caring for dying residents. The interactions between these two groups influence practical decisions regarding the site and nature of care for dying residents (Katz *et al.* 1999).

Few studies have investigated the roles of the primary health care team and specialist palliative nurses in relation to residents dying in care settings. This chapter therefore heavily relies on the data collected in the two OU Studies and data from Froggatt's survey of clinical nurse specialists in palliative care (2001) and their relationships with care homes. In the two OU Studies the views of external health workers were sought through interviews or workshops about the nature of their work with dying people in residential settings; in addition a perspective on their contribution to these decisions were provided by home managers, other home staff, relatives, and colleagues from other disciplines.

The role of the general practitioner

Family doctors in providing medical supervision influence or determine the nature of care and site of death of people dying in care homes. This can sometimes explain (a) decisions over whether dying people are transferred to hospital or another setting and (b) a reluctance or alternatively a willingness to retain dying residents in the homes. The latter means GPs taking responsibility for addressing their 'total care' needs.

To date there is very little documented data on the attitudes of general practitioners to caring for people dying in residential care and nursing home settings. However, there are at least four relevant studies which report GPs' accounts of caring for dying and bereaved people in the community (Field 1998; Harris and Kendrick 1998; Higginson 1999; Saunderson and Ridsdale 1999). Higginson (1999) using survey methodology ascertained the views of GPs on local specialist palliative care services. Field followed a cohort of medical students who graduated in 1979 and then worked in general practice. He explored their attitudes towards caring for people dying in community settings. Like the OU Study (1) Field explored definitions of dying and perceptions of the appropriateness of palliative care for people dying of non-malignant disease. Using similar qualitative methodology Saunderson and Ridsdale (1999) have conducted semi-structured interviews with GPs followed by a qualitative content analysis. They focused on GPs perceptions of their effectiveness in relation to bereaved relatives. In particular they explored how GPs felt about their skills in relation to medical practice when patients died and whether they experienced feelings of guilt and loss. Harris and Kendrick (1998) acknowledging that bereavement support has been advocated as an area of prevention in primary care explored GPs perceptions and action taken by them following patient death notifications by hospitals and hospices. These four studies demonstrate the challenges faced by GPs in managing dying peoples' care.

In OU Study (1) 22 GPs were interviewed to ascertain their views about appropriate terminal care for people dying in care settings. Two of these GPs no longer worked in conventional practices, but in local hospices. The remaining 20 GPs were responsible for the care of specific residents who died in the homes during the study period. They ranged in age from early thirties till late sixties; the sample therefore included some GPs who had received some training in palliative medicine in medical school. Data from this study, albeit small, inform this chapter.

Three fundamental issues determined how these GPs evaluated terminal care in care settings. The first related to their perceptions of their responsibilities towards and relationships with care homes; the second was their perception of the nature of the dying trajectory of older people dying in residential settings; the third was their understanding of the principles and practices of palliative care and its relevance to older people.

GPs relationships with homes

Looking after 'patients' in residential or nursing homes can constitute a substantial proportion of GPs workloads. With the de-institutionalization of long-stay NHS wards, where older people were nursed within the hospital, many GPs have found their workload has increased (Barclay 2001). The GPs often are associated with several homes and conversely some homes are visited by many practices. In OU Study (1) five of the 100 home managers reported that 12 practices served their homes (Komaromy *et al.* 2000). This means that carers have to develop working relationships with at least several primary health teams. However within group practices, one GP tended to take the responsibility for most of the practice's 'patients' in each individual home. It was relatively rare for residents to retain their 'own' GPs following admission to a nursing or residential care home.

Most GPs were positive about the way in which most home managers used their services and did not differentiate between nursing and residential care homes in this regard. Although they noted an increase in their 'geriatric workload' they did not attribute this to inappropriate demands made on their time, but rather to demographic changes, with people living longer and more likely to spend their old and frail years in residential care. GPs who had a high proportion of their patients resident in homes reported a good working relationship with the homes.

GPs views about appropriate terminal care in care homes

GPs differentiated between terminal care in domestic settings as opposed to nursing and residential care homes (Katz *et al.* 1999). They valued the contribution community nurses could make to caring for people dying in their own homes, particularly their role in setting up and supervising the use of syringe drivers (Goodman *et al.* 1998). Most GPs in the OU Study did not feel that either residential or nursing homes should or could manage pain control which needed to be delivered through a syringe driver (pump). Indeed one GP quoted a myth popular in one geographical area in which the study took place that homes which were not registered to deliver nursing care (i.e. residential homes) were not allowed by law to set up syringe drivers. This myth was shared by some home managers as well as some community nurses.

Only 3 of the 20 GPs had ever agreed to a syringe driver being set up in a residential home (Katz et al. 1999), and only then because they perceived the dying person to be in intractable pain; they would not consider this as a normal pain control measure. 'Prescribing' a syringe driver depended on first their assessment of the quality and dependability of the care staff in the home to provide physical care and second their confidence in the community nurses to set up and supervise the use of the syringe driver.

GPs shared a common vision of what constituted good terminal care in residential and nursing homes. When comparing different establishments their views about terminal care were expressed almost exclusively in terms of recognizing and addressing physical symptoms. For example one GP noted with concern that in one home, staff reported finding a resident's moaning irritating rather than acknowledging that this could be an indication that the resident was in pain. Another noted:

> I think they need to know how to look out for pain. Sometimes I've gone in to see a patient and you know that they're in pain. They can't actually say 'ouch, it hurts', but you can read the lines on their face. Pain is something that can be seen and felt in the face. When you're moving a patient, the tension.

However GPs' perceptions of appropriate end-of-life care in care homes was closely linked to their perceptions of the needs of older people and their views about palliative care.

GPs understandings of palliative care for older people

The primary workload of general practitioners is with people of all ages living more or less independently in their own homes. Consequently their most frequent contact with dying people is with those dying in their own homes, under the care of hospital physicians (and/or a hospital based palliative care team) and who may be looked after by the local hospice, Macmillan nurse, or palliative care team. Usually people dying in their own homes are likely to be dying of an acute illness and younger than the average population living in care homes. It is important to remember that this is the norm GPs associate when thinking about palliative care.

A number of studies have explored doctors' perceptions of palliative care (summarized in Barclay 2001). This resembles the perceptions of the host population, that palliative care, or hospice involvement is most appropriate for younger people living at home and dying of cancer. In OU Study (1) most GPs saw palliative care as synonymous with *pain and symptom control for*

cancer and had its place, either in the hospice under the guidance of a palliative care physician or in the domestic arena with community nurses advised by
Macmillan nurses (Katz *et al.* 1999). They never considered the possibility that
palliative care *services* could be appropriate for adults suffering from
non-malignant disease (Addington-Hall 1998).

In the OU Study (1), GPs differentiated between the dying trajectories of
younger and older people. In their view, palliative care was inappropriate for
older people for a variety of reasons. First they suggested that older people
experience a gradual deterioration in their health. Second GPs believed that
symptom and pain control is fairly straightforward to manage in this population. Third, several GPs presenting themselves as their patients' advocates, suggested that older people do not favour intervention, such as drips and suctions.
This was a very frequently expressed common sense assumption based on
their experience, rather than on any collected documentation and often
expressed in words approximating the following: '*Older people did not actively
want to live or die, they just fade away*'

> What often happens in many nursing homes patients get very elderly, they get very
> frail. And I think pain control is possibly not always so difficult, it is much more
> significant for the younger patients. We get on to oral analgesia and then injections
> would be catered for. I think if we needed something more sophisticated, syringe
> drivers or more complicated care, they would be off to a hospice certainly.

The quote above suggests that this GP might refer a resident to a hospice. Yet
as OU Study (1) indicated (see Chapter 3), dying residents were not conventional candidates for admission to a hospice at least in terms of the conditions
from which they suffered. But many older people in this study experienced
complicated symptoms that were hard to control such as painful spasms from
Parkinson's Disease and muscular sclerosis.

When questioned about pain control in relation to non-malignant conditions, half the GPs saw this as problematic especially where older people were
dying from heart failure or conditions other than cancer. An unusual GP who
believed that the type of analgesia should not be determined by the nature of
the underlying disease noted that:

> Very often doctors are too reluctant to slap up their analgesia. A lot of doctors
> seem to reserve it for cancer patients and nobody else. And I think that's wrong.
> Anybody who has an incurable chronic painful complaint deserves to have
> adequate analgesia. . . my colleagues looked quite askance at me for using
> morphine for an old lady who had severe osteo-arthritis of the back.

Many GPs echoed the views of home staff that morphine was not an appropriate drug to prescribe for older people. They used morphine and related

analgesia conservatively maintaining that it was appropriate for end stage malignant conditions. A hospice doctor explained why:

> A lot of GPs are frightened of using (morphine) because they've not had a recent lecture about it. (Where they do use MST) many of them tend to use very small doses and don't increase it to the right levels.

Familiarity with pharmacological preparations is hard to measure in qualitative studies. GPs in the United Kingdom receive quantities of literature about medication from the Department of Health and from drug companies, and they find it hard to keep up to date in this area. The WHO analgesic ladder for pain control has been available for more than a decade and an assumption might be made that as pain control is likely to be a fairly important element of general practice, most GPs would be familiar with this. However in OU Study (1) only three GPs were fairly familiar with the analgesic ladder and were able to explain the logic of progressive analgesia:

> I started off with oramorph because it's one you can increase and decrease the dose. Then we went straight to MST, 20 milligrams in suspension because you can give that as a liquid . . . She was certainly in pain so she was given MST because it was going to keep her (a) comfortable and (b) shorten the duration of any discomfort that she would have in her death.

Only a few GPs acknowledged that syringe drivers could contain medication to relieve not only cancer related pain, but also vomiting and malabsorption as well as symptoms caused by cardiac failure. One GP spoke about giving terminally ill patients an anti-nausea drug as well which also had a sedating effect.

Familiarity with concept of total pain

The concept of total pain was coined by Dame Cecily Saunders (in Saunders and Sykes 1993) to include physical, social, emotional, psychological, and spiritual components of pain. This comprehensive description of how pain can be experienced is the cornerstone upon which palliative care is based. It is self-evident that in order to address these five elements, doctors will require good communication skills particularly in relation to older people some of whom will have lost the ability to communicate in conventional ways. Five of the 22 GPs interviewed understood that the concept of total pain included emotional and spiritual elements:

> Her medical needs were pain relief and psychological boosting, backup, and reassurance. I think she was very frightened. And the lymphodema frightened her quite a lot.

Few GPs in the OU Study raised 'communication' per se as an integral part of terminal care. However several issues in relation to communication emerged. None of the GPs believed that it was appropriate to talk to residents about dying. The explanation given was that older people accept the inevitability of death. Only one GP spoke about involving a dying resident in the decision of whether to admit her to hospital and even in this case, this decision turned on medical grounds. In contrast to Flacker *et al.* (2001) where family physicians expressed concern about the amount of emotional support they were providing to relatives, GPs in the OU Study (1) did not see communicating with relatives as an important aspect of caring for dying residents.

Only one (Muslim) GP expressed concern about spiritual needs:

> When people are about to die, they remember their whole lives, their own existence, their creation, creator, all kinds of things. And I think in this era of so-called scientific progress, that has been very neglected, or imposed upon the patient, according to the will of the establishment they're in . . . I think in Western countries, people are afraid of talking about religion, or God, or things like that. Very much afraid. And they think that even by saying so they will offend the person. But maybe sometimes a patient wants it. Because he or she is dying, losing the connection with this life, and this world, they want to know.

Communication with dying people is an ongoing process from initial contact with the dying person and their informal (and/or paid) carers through the whole dying trajectory. Bereavement care is central to the teamwork espoused in the principles of palliative care and the primary care team not only experience some grief themselves but also have some responsibility for acknowledging the grief of those left behind. Although bereavement care was seen as a developing area in GPs workload and prompted the study by Harris and Kendrick (1998) they found that only 39 per cent of the practices they surveyed routinely offered bereaved relatives support from a member of the primary care health team. Thirty-eight per cent of the 353 GPs surveyed noted that they only supported relatives who asked for help. GPs in the OU Study (1) did not conceptualize bereavement care with deceased residents' relatives as part of their particular remit. In relation to care homes, not only are relatives bereft, but care staff also grieve when residents die, and this might be an area that GPs engage in, even in a very limited way.

Discussion

Barclay (2001) notes that three particular elements make the primary care team the obvious choice for providing palliative care in the community, and two of these elements are pertinent to care homes. First, quoting Field (1998)

Barclay notes that GPs believe in the *continuity* of patient care, which is not possible in the hospital sector. GPs are able to establish relationships over time with patients and their families (and formal carers in the instance of care homes). A long-term relationship is not feasible for specialist palliative care teams, although as noted elsewhere in the book there is a movement towards involving these teams much earlier on in the illness, so that the relationship is not one of crisis intervention. Second, central to the primary health care team is the concept of *multi-disciplinarity*, a fundamental feature of palliative care. Barclay quotes the study of Kurti and O'Dowd (1995) where GPs and community nurses identified the team approach as the 'most important aspect of their palliative care provision' and this was also emphasized by GPs in the OU Study (1). Barclay (2001) also cites Grande's research which focused on ways in which GPs and community nurses are able to complement one another's skills in providing palliative care. (The third relates to the family perspective which, although often relevant in relation to residents in care homes, their family members may predecease them or live at a distance.)

GPs should not expect to provide palliative care without the support of other agencies and also have to cope emotionally with distressed dying people and their carers. For GPs dealing with increased workloads and the changing nature of general practice, providing supportive palliative care in care homes is not going to be any more straightforward than it is at present. In addition, educational strategies in palliative care for GPs will need to reflect their needs and preferences (Shipman *et al.* 2001).

Community (District) nurses

Community nurses, also known as district nurses in the United Kingdom, provide nursing services to people living in their own homes and also in non-hospital institutional settings. Although they are employed by the community National Health Service trusts they provide care for the patients served by specific general practices in their own homes and residential homes. Whether this will change with the new regulation of care homes is not yet clear (see Chapter 2). Prior to community care legislation in the early 1990s the work of community nurses included a mixture of health and personal care such as bathing, changing dressings and a variety of specialized nursing 'treatments'; in more recent years the personal aspects of this care in private domestic settings has been funded by social services and provided by health care assistants. In residential homes, the personal aspects of care is provided by care staff working in the home, and community nurses primarily provide 'expert nursing care'.

As Seale noted in 1992, community nurses deliver more terminal and palliative nursing care than any other group of health workers. Not only do they do hands-on care, but they provide advice and counselling to dying people and their families. It is an area of their work from which they derive considerable satisfaction (Goodman *et al.* 1998). As 'dying at home' has become more acceptable both to the lay population and health care workers, community nurses are increasingly familiar and comfortable supporting families to deliver analgesia. Skills possessed by community nurses are easily transferable into different settings—for example, their knowledge and familiarity with analgesia could be put to just as good use in care homes as in the private domestic setting (OU Study (1)). In residential care, community nurses are the linchpin of health care relationships for residents and their families and a community nurse could be providing hands-on care for many years to an individual resident before that resident is necessarily defined as 'dying'.

But what is the structural position of external nursing staff and how could they support staff in care homes to develop planned and sustained palliative care plans for dying residents? (This issue is further discussed in Chapter 11 by Field and Froggatt.) *Nursing* homes by law are obliged to have a trained nurse on duty at all times and rarely call upon the services of community nurses. However the 12 community nurses interviewed in the OU Study (1) felt that they could make a considerable contribution to caring for dying people in *nursing* homes and were willing to extend their case load to do so. In many instances community nurses assumed that the quality of terminal care provided by *nursing* homes was poor and noted that, for example, very few *nursing* homes possessed syringe drivers nor knew how to operate them. Community nurses recognized that one of their own strengths was their regular updating which placed them in a strong position to teach staff working in both *nursing* homes and *residential* homes and they welcomed this role. Similar to the findings in the Avis *et al.* (1999) study, OU Study (1) found that nurses employed in nursing homes had few opportunities to keep abreast of new developments:

> Nurses are very out of date in nursing homes—they don't do catheterization, a lot of them don't do bloods, a lot don't do syringe drivers. They should keep themselves up to date and we're hoping that perhaps they will improve. The girls in nursing homes have said that they don't (update themselves) because the owners of the homes say it's up to the girls to do it themselves and they must pay. And a lot of these girls are paid very low hourly rates and they can't afford it.

Avis *et al.* (1999) have reported on an evaluation of a pilot project that sought to improve the provision of palliative care support to nursing homes. They have found that nursing home staff felt less isolated following the input of community nurses who were providing a palliative care service. Additionally, the project decreased the inequity of access to specialist palliative care services for nursing home residents.

Relationship with home

In OU Study (1) community nurses were used by all the *residential* homes on a regular basis. They visited residents (referred to them by the GPs to whom they were attached) for a variety of nursing needs, mostly unconnected with terminal care. Observational findings from case study homes indicated that often community nurses did not engage particularly with care staff, only visiting their 'patients' to carry out particular functions such as changing dressings.

The roles played by community nurses in residential homes depended on their relationship with home managers. Where the home manager was a qualified nurse, community nurses felt more confident about the home's ability to assess a resident. However, even when this was not the case community nurses often felt that they were used sensibly and that they had a good relationship with care staff.

When a resident was deteriorating, providing terminal care presented a dilemma and challenge for the home staff. Home managers regarded community nurses as an essential resource primarily in relation to supporting them to provide physical care, which they equated with terminal care. For example, community nurses provided two crucial components of practical physical support, first supplying mattresses and other equipment and second in relation to providing specialist care such as attending to pressure areas or setting up syringe drivers.

Community nurses believe that they should become involved early in the care of ill residents long before the resident is defined as 'dying' (OU Study (1); Barclay *et al.* 1999; Luker *et al.* 2000). This involvement should include contact with the patient and family, establishing continuity of care, spending time with the dying person and providing more than simply physical care (Luker *et al.* 2000). Forty-eight per cent of community nurses in Seale's (1992) study felt that GPs referred the patient too late to develop a meaningful and trusting relationship.

Without this early involvement the work of community nurses becomes crisis intervention (OU Study (1)), rather than preventative and/or longstanding. Community nurses complained that carers in residential homes endeavoured to manage the situation themselves too long and only called community nurses when things deteriorated (OU Study (1)). Earlier intervention on their part could have prevented problems such as the development of pressure sores. Additionally they noted that they were not given sufficient information about either the condition or what the dying person or family knew about the diagnosis.

Whilst home managers in OU Study (1) saw community nurses as providing a limited service, community nurses thought their role should be multidimensional and identified the following components: assessment leading to a care plan; supply of appropriate aids and education and emotional support of care staff and liasing with the GPs.

Assessment and use of care plans

Community nurses interviewed in the OU Study (1) stressed that when they were referred a terminally ill resident, they first undertook an assessment and then developed a care plan. The assessment included how often a patient needed visiting, particularly if the patient had a syringe driver. This included making contact with specialist palliative care services if necessary, for example, enquiring about dosages and symptom control, or referring patients to other specialist services, for example, a stroke nurse. Community nurses noted that even in nursing homes, care plans are not always used. In residential homes community nurses had to convince the staff of their usefulness when caring for a dying resident. The way in which home staff understand their roles is crucial to good care.

Education and supporting roles

The educational aspects of community nurses' roles included practical hands on teaching, trying to teach carers basic skills such as pain awareness, and helping them to become more confident in caring for dying residents (OU Study (1)). As residential workers were not regularly accustomed to managing syringe drivers, community nurses had to explain how they operate and what to do if they stopped working. But there was much more basic teaching to do, for example, simple lifting techniques, suggestions about diet, as well as explaining the principles behind whole person care:

> They have got to be able to look at the whole person . . . when a patient is dying there are all sorts of things other than the obvious illness . . . I would like to think that the carers were aware of other things that happen to the patient, the other bodily functions and anything involved in the comfort. Even though the patient might say she doesn't want a drink she still needs her mouth taken care of—oral hygiene.

Very often the community nurse becomes the main external contact for end-stage non-malignant disease (Barclay 2001). The educational role of community nurses might therefore encompass teaching care staff aspects of palliative care for residents not suffering from malignant conditions:

> We go into the home and advise on palliative care for conditions other than cancer. Patients with chest problems for instance. There are ways of controlling the symptoms, positions, medication (the GP would probably be involved).

> Symptom control for stroke patients. The stroke patient is often very agitated in some ways and there again that symptom can be controlled—it just requires a very small amount of medication. So if we go in and see the symptoms then quite often we do then liase with the GP.

Community nurses noted that they also provided emotional support for carers:

> We play a big part in supporting staff. I find that when they (staff) are not from a nursing background, they're very apprehensive about death and dying. And sometimes you've got to talk through the stages and what can happen. Sometimes (we're here) just for the staff to off load. They get very involved with them and sometimes they can't be objective. I think sometimes they worry that they're not meeting the needs and they're doing everything that they possibly can and they need a lot of reassurance. They worry if their needs change—but they always have a contact number and we'll come straight away if there's a change.

Supporting home staff to keep a dying person in the home also included acknowledging the additional burden this care placed on already over-stretched carers who might feel that transferring the resident to hospital might be the best option (OU Study (1)). Therefore community nurses are some-times implicated in the decisions to transfer residents, and have to maintain the delicate balance of supporting care workers to keep the resident without making carers feel threatened by their (superior) expertise.

> I always discuss the ability of the staff to have this extra workload and be able to care for them. If it's a short-term situation I would say it's unfair to move her to a nursing home. But if it's a long term thing and you can't always tell then we have the question of whether this patient is in the right place for him or her. And that's where we run into difficulties. Residential homes are quite reluctant to let their patients go, and it's not always the staff, it's the families, they don't want them moved. The patient may have been there for a number of years they've got to know the staff. It may be financial, it's going to cost twice as much in a nursing home.

Relationships with GPs

Decisions about transferring a resident and the management of medication in care homes can generate conflict between community nurses and GPs. In OU Study (1), those community nurses who reported a good relationship with their GPs were able to persuade them to set up, or allow them to install syringe drivers in some *residential* homes. However even when they were up and run-ning community nurses reported that sometimes GPs confused the situation by changing the rate inappropriately. In addition, they suggested that GPs occasionally lacked understanding about the nature of the high quality nurs-ing care required to care for dying residents. Similar to findings in the study conducted by Avis *et al.* (1999) community nurses noted that not only did GPs lack basic knowledge about palliative care but they also misjudged the capabilities of home staff:

> Quite often the doctors will be visiting a patient who goes on to develop bronchitis and they naturally think the staff can cope with that. And they don't because quite often the complications of bed rest follow on. I went in to see this chap who'd had the flu and he had blisters all along his feet. And the senior care worker said 'Oh dear, he's only been in bed 48 hours'. And that is a complete lack of understanding of somebody with, chest infection, debilitated, not eating, on bed rest 48 hours, why would they have a pressure sore. Whereas a trained nurse hopefully would understand that as soon as they're in that state they need to go into preventive care.

Discussion

The role of community nurses in providing palliative care not only depends on the factors raised above, but also on their access to resources which depends partly on the nature of the dying person's illness. Someone dying of cancer has more access to resources, for example, specialist palliative care team, Marie Curie sitters, or respite care than someone of heart failure. However, community nurses interviewed in OU Study (1) noted that families and carers often face the same problems regardless of the diagnosis.

The 12 community nurses interviewed felt that their own expertise in palliative care was sufficient and had not brought in specialist palliative care nurses for advice, although they assumed that such specialists were called into *residential* homes by home staff or referred by GPs. It was difficult to assess whether community nurses interacted at all with specialist palliative care nurses as contact was only mentioned in relation to attending training sessions (Katz *et al.* 1999). However, one might safely assume from the findings of Austin *et al.* (2000) that along with other cited conditions for high quality palliative care the relationship with other healthcare professionals as well as informal carers are very important factors.

Community nurses see palliative care as an ideal type of nursing to which all other areas of nursing might aspire, 'an exemplar of excellence' (Goodman *et al.* 1998; Luker *et al.* 2000) and welcome opportunities to engage in delivering nursing care in a way that has been eroded in other areas through the redefinitions of the community nursing service.

Specialist palliative care teams

There is very little documented information in the United Kingdom about the roles played by specialist palliative care teams in relation to caring for residents dying in care homes other than the recent survey of clinical nurse specialists

(CNS) undertaken by Froggatt *et al.* (2001). Their study found that although community palliative clinical nurse specialists had considerable contact with nursing homes and less contact with residential homes there was no sustained relationship, contacts were 'infrequent and reactive and focuses primarily on direct clinical work' (p. 22). As would be expected CNSs were rarely consulted in relation to non-malignant conditions, and they responded to referrals rather than initiating contact themselves. The small number of Macmillan nurses interviewed in the OU Study (1) several years earlier suggested that they too were used on an *ad hoc* basis, but very rarely in both nursing and residential homes (Katz *et al.* 1999). Like respondents in Froggatt's study they felt that the lack of their involvement mostly related to misconceptions about their roles and their skills in the wider society which they believed was shared by home managers and GPs. Froggatt's respondents were however able to undertake some education and training in care settings, particularly in nursing homes where they could more easily interact with the nominated link-nurse.

A hospice doctor interviewed for the OU Study (1) suggested that residents died in uncontrolled pain or were unnecessarily transferred to die in hospital simply because of the ignorance about the service that specialist palliative care teams could offer. This situation is not unique to the United Kingdom. Data from the United States suggest similarly that hospice care is also not making the appropriate inroads into nursing homes and this absence contributes to the poor end-of-life care received by dying nursing home residents (Keay and Schonwetter 2000). However, as Chapter 10 indicates, the situation in the United States is more complex than in the United Kingdom because of the way hospice care is funded. The logical assumption would be that nursing and residential homes in the United Kingdom should have easier access to all the services, both hands-on care, advice, and education that specialist palliative care offers precisely because hospice provision is free at the point of delivery.

Conclusion

From the little data available, it is apparent that one of the main stumbling blocks to seamless palliative care in care settings is the lack of cohesiveness between the service providers. In the United Kingdom the relationship between palliative care teams and primary health care teams working in care homes is *ad hoc* without financial agreements. In an Australian study where palliative care nurses working in three settings of care (community, hospice, and hospital) were asked to describe communication issues for an interdisciplinary community palliative care, the team reported that there were a number of issues which prevented satisfactory communication between palliative care nurses and GPs. These included networking, case management, multiple service providers, lack of standardized documentation and formal teaching of clients, along with difficulties in transmission of relevant practice knowledge (Street and Blackford 2001). All of these issues seem to be quite pertinent to the care home setting in the United Kingdom which in itself does not provide a standardized service.

In conclusion, interdisciplinary co-operation centring around the needs of a dying resident would benefit all the parties and should focus on encouraging those from different disciplines to work together. A multidisciplinary team is only a team if they negotiate their roles and ensure seamless care (Street and Blackford 2001; and see Chapter 11). Carers in residential and nursing home settings would benefit from the support of palliative care teams particularly if constructive communication takes place between care staff, the primary care team, and specialist palliative care services.

References

Addington-Hall, J. (1998) *Reaching out: Specialist Palliative Care for Adults with Non-malignant Diseases*. National Council for Hospice and Specialist Palliative Care Services and Scottish Partnership Agency for Palliative and Cancer Care.

Austin, L., Luker, K.A., Caress, A., and Hallett, C.E. (2000) Palliative care: Community nurses' perceptions of quality. *Quality in Health Care*, 9(3), 151–8.

Avis, M., Jackson, J.G., Cox, K., and Miskella, C. (1999) Evaluation of a project providing community palliative care support to nursing homes. *Health and Social Care in the Community*, 7(1), 32–8.

Barclay, S., Todd, C., McCabe, J., and Hunt, T. (1999) Primary care group commissioning of services: The differing priorities of general practitioners and district nurses for palliative care services. *British Journal of General Practice*, 49(440), 181–6.

Barclay, S. (2001) A UK perspective from primary care, in J.M. Addington-Hall and I.J. Higginson (eds) *Palliative Care for Non-Cancer Patients*. Oxford University Press, Oxford.

Field, D. (1998) Special, not different: General practitioners' accounts of their care of dying people. *Social Science and Medicine*, 46(9), 1111–20.

Flacker, J.M., Won, A., Kiely, D.K., and Iloputaife, I. (2001) Differing perceptions of end-of-life care in long-term care. *Journal of Palliative Medicine*, 4(1), 9–13.

Froggatt, K., Hoult, L., and Poole, K. (2001) *Community Work with Nursing and Residential Care Homes: A Survey Study of Clinical Nurse Specialists in Palliative Care*. Macmillan Cancer Relief, London.

Goodman, C., Knight, D., Machen, I., and Hunt, B. (1998) Emphasizing terminal care as district nursing work: A helpful strategy in a purchasing environment? *Journal of Advanced Nursing*, 28(3), 491–8.

Harris, T. and Kendrick, T. (1998) Bereavement care in general practice: A survey in South Thames Health Region. *The British Journal of General Practice: the Journal of the Royal College of General Practitioners*, 48(434), 1560–4.

Higginson, I. (1999) Palliative care services in the community: What do family doctors want? *Journal of Palliative Care*, **15**(2), 21–5.

Katz, J.T., Komaromy, C., and Sidell, M. (1999) Understanding palliative care in residential and nursing homes. *International Journal of Palliative Nursing*, **5**(2), 58–64.

Keay, T.J. and Schonwetter, R.S. (2000) The case for hospice care in long-term environments. *Clinics in Geriatric Medicine*, **16**(2), 211–23.

Kurti, I. and O'Dowd, T. (1995) Dying of non malignant diseases in general practice. *Journal of Palliative Care*, **11**(3), 25–31.

Luker, K.A., Austin, L., Caress, A., and Hallett, C.E. (2000) The importance of 'knowing the patient': community nurses' constructions of quality in providing palliative care. *Journal of Advanced Nursing*, **31**(4), 775–82.

Saunders, C. and Sykes, N. (1993) *The Management of Terminal Illness* (3rd edition). Edward Arnold, London.

Saunderson, E.M. and Ridsdale, L. (1999) General practitioners' beliefs and attitudes about how to respond to death and bereavement: qualitative study. *BMJ* **319**, 293–6.

Seale, C. (1992) Community nurses and the care of the dying. *Social Science and Medicine*, **34**(4), 375–82.

Shipman, C., Addington-Hall, J., Barclay, S., Briggs, J., Cox, I., Daniels, L., and Millar, D. (2001) Educational opportunities in palliative care: What do general practitioners want? *Palliative Medicine*, **15**, 191–6.

Street, A. and Blackford, J. (2001) Communication issues for the interdisciplinary community palliative care team. *Journal of Clinical Nursing*, **10**(5), 643–50.

Chapter 8

The training needs of carers

Moyra Sidell

Introduction

Previous chapters have documented the fact that residential and nursing homes provide terminal care for large numbers of older people. These numbers are likely to increase as recent policies in continuing care have meant that more older people are cared for outside of the hospital setting. Yet staff in these settings care for their dying residents with very little training or guidance (Dalley and Denniss 2001). This situation gives cause for concern both for the quality of care provided for dying older people and the attendant stresses on staff in homes. The lack of nationwide training in this area has made the provision of terminal care for older people in these settings an urgent matter. Much of this chapter is based on the OU Studies referred to in Chapter 1. It will draw mainly on OU Study (2) which developed and tested a set of training materials tailored to the needs of care workers and all those involved in caring for dying people in care homes (see Chapter 1: p. 9). The first section of this chapter focuses on establishing the need for training to improve the quality of terminal care available to dying residents. It argues that training in the basic principles and practices of palliative care is one, but not the only factor, that has the potential to improve the quality of dying in care homes. In order to create a culture which can help people to express their hopes and fears about death and dying it is important that training should target all levels of staff and that the training should be appropriate to their needs. The following section addresses this question of who needs training and then goes on to explore the level of knowledge and skills needed by different types of staff and reviews the development of appropriate training materials. The final section returns to the issue that training alone will not necessarily improve the quality of dying in care homes and puts training in the wider context of resources and explores the conditions needed to enable training to flourish.

Why train?

The document 'Modernising the Social Care Workforce' (TOPSS 1999) expressed concern about an unqualified workforce in which 80 per cent of all social care staff are without formal qualification. The government document 'Fit for the Future' (DoH 1999) recommended that older people who live in residential and nursing home settings should receive a better quality of care that is based on the principles of dignity, choice, privacy, and respect and National Minimum Standards for Care Homes for Older People have been set based on these key principles (DoH 2001) with the expectation that at least 50 per cent of care assistants in homes should be trained to NVQ Level two by 2005. As seen in Chapter 2 (pp. 37–8) Standard 11 focuses on death and dying stating that it is a requirement that: '*Care and comfort are given to service users who are dying, their death is handled with dignity and propriety, and their spiritual needs, rites and functions observed*' (DoH 2001: 13). The ability of homes to implement this standard specifically in relation to terminal care is dependent upon home staff being trained in the relevant areas.

The care of dying people has developed into a specialized activity with a set of principles and practices. Specialist care is carried out by highly trained professionals working primarily in hospices, palliative care domiciliary teams (and Macmillan nurses), and some hospitals. As noted in Chapter 3, 83 per cent of deaths now occur in old age (Office of National Statistics 1999) and 18 per cent of these deaths take place in care homes (Froggatt 2000). Thus much of the care of dying older people takes place in these settings. At present the terminal care provided particularly in residential but also in nursing homes is largely undertaken by unqualified staff, most of whom have had no training in the care of dying or bereaved people. Training was identified in a study carried out by Counsel and Care (1995) as an area, where there were 'significant gaps'. And another small study concluded that staff need 'training coupled with support' otherwise 'residents and staff alike may suffer adversely' (Shemmings 1996: 102). A more recent nationwide study carried out by the Centre for Policy on Ageing (Dalley and Denniss 2001) found that only a very small amount (just 3 per cent on bereavement care) of the training that is undertaken in care homes is devoted to issues directly relevant to terminal care. The OU Study (1) also found that other professionals who visit the homes on an *ad hoc* basis often lack specialized training in these areas. Training is then an urgent area of concern. As Dalley and Denniss (2001) found apart from some statutory training requirements, and, in England, some NVQ training in a small number of homes which has some relevance to the care of dying people, care staff carry out these sensitive tasks with little or no guidance.

The OU Study (1) found that care staff felt very strongly that residents should be allowed to die in familiar surroundings in what had become their last home (see Chapters 3 and 4). They frequently articulated the needs of residents who were dying in terms of pain relief and dignity, as one registered manager put it:

> Well I should think it is just to make sure the patient dies without pain, maintains their control and dignity up until the end.

But many registered managers felt unsure of their own ability to provide the necessary care and the continued failure to recognize a longer dying trajectory discussed in Chapter 3 of this book means that the residents' needs for terminal care is limited to the last few days of their lives. As noted in Chapter 4 only a third of the registered managers interviewed in OU Study (1) had any understanding of the palliative care approach. It was also clear that many homes have little or no training budget, and minimal staff cover does not allow for the release of staff for training. The findings were very much in line with the Dalley and Denniss study (2001) in that existing training in homes is disparate and of a variable standard. The training initiatives that do exist, range from short sessions for care assistants, usually on bereavement and loss, to more technical training for qualified nurses. Staff with actual qualifications in palliative care are a rarity. OU Study (1) revealed very little training either in house or attendance on courses which were specifically about the care of dying and bereaved people. Many homes said they were involved with NVQ training but the majority of this did not include death and dying and we had little evidence of staff completing courses. Some homes talked about informal training such as taking the opportunity to discuss issues of death and dying as and when they arose. But compared to training in lifting, management of pressure sores, death, and dying was conspicuous by its absence.

A key finding of OU Study (1) was that:

> Knowledge of palliative care philosophy and techniques was rare, often it was oversimplified and limited or else seen as highly technical and inappropriate. This limited view seriously impairs the ability of the heads of homes to judge the adequacy of care given to their dying residents. There exists a complacency borne of lack of vision. Goodwill is in abundance, knowledge and expertise is sadly lacking. Very few staff had any palliative care qualifications and this was reflected in their lack of understanding of palliative care concepts.
>
> (Sidell *et al.* 1997: ix)

Another source of information on the need of home staff for training in terminal care came from interviews with external supporters to the homes, particularly community and Macmillan nurses. A specialist palliative care nurse who provided support to one of the homes we worked in was convinced that home staff need training in all aspects of palliative care and that this should not be specifically geared to patients with cancer. She said:

> Just because a patient hasn't got cancer and maybe has had a stroke or may be at the end stage of another disease does not mean that they should be treated differently from somebody with cancer. So they need training in all aspects of palliative care so that they can use it as a general approach to all their clientele not specifically the patients that we are involved in.

Macmillan nurses were acutely aware of the lack of skills of home staff in recognizing pain, one said:

> A common scenario is that the patient is reported to be pain free. And then when we visit them, the patient is rigid in bed. We have to explain gently that the patient may not appear to have any pain but when they're moved, then their medication needs adjusting accordingly. And also getting them to recognise these different sorts of pain; pain caused from tumour problems, pain caused from hernia problems and even psychological pain.

OU Study (1) strongly recommended:

> Education and training for all staff so that they have a deeper understanding of the principles and practice of palliative care. Training would also need to address the issue of defining dying in older people whose dying trajectory is likely to be different from those dying of cancer. Recognising the need for palliative care much earlier in the dying trajectory than the last few days of life would allow for much more effective pain relief and symptom control.
>
> (Sidell *et al.* 1997: xii)

In 1997 Macmillan Cancer Relief and the Wolfson Foundation funded a two-year pilot training project for 400 care assistants working in nursing homes in Cheshire (Smith 1998). This was evaluated by Katherine Froggatt (2000). She looked at the impact of the training on the care of residents and their families. She found that the training had most impact in the area of pain control and that the knowledge gained benefited other residents and not only those who were said to be dying. Other benefits were noted in communication with residents in that care staff felt more willing and able to listen to residents and talk about difficult issues surrounding death and dying. A greater awareness was also developed in understanding the needs of family and friends and of other staff in times of loss. A reservation discussed by Froggatt (2001) was the limited impact of training on the 'culture' of a home which she identified as an important factor in the quality of terminal care (see Chapters 2, 11, and 12). It is however important to note that the study she evaluated provided educational courses in palliative care separately to three different groups of staff, registered nurses, healthcare assistants, and ancilliary staff. OU Study (2) found that it was vital that all levels of staff should take part in training programmes together and that getting the registered managers involved in the actual training was the key to changing the culture of the home (Katz *et al*. 2000). The staff composition on training programmes has an important effect on the learning experience but also on the wider impact on the home.

Who needs training?

The model of sending selected members of staff on training courses is of limited benefit in terms of changing the way that the home as a whole deals with death and dying. We found that all levels of staff in homes can be involved to a greater or lesser degree when someone is dying or has died. Kitchen staff, domestic staff, and gardeners although not directly involved in care nevertheless interact with all the residents and over what is often a period of years can build up quite strong attachments. They may be approached for information or just to talk about someone's fears and they will probably have got to know relatives and friends well. Care assistants are directly involved in the day to day care of residents when they are dying and are often in a prime position to discuss residents' feelings and fears. They are also in a good position to assess the level of pain that a resident might be experiencing. OU Study (2) argued strongly that staff at all levels in homes need some training in how to deal with death and dying.

It was felt essential that any training materials should be used in-house and with groups of staff at all levels working together. There were several reasons for this. The first reason was that if all groups of staff work together in groups in the homes they can draw on their collective experiences, share their knowledge and skills and identify areas of strengths as well as weaknesses and negotiate areas for change. The training is more likely to have an impact on the care of dying residents in the home because all levels of staff will be committed to their learning and to the need for change. However the issue of whether the registered managers should attend did give rise to some problems.

Registered manager's involvement

Registered managers attended most of the developmental training workshops in OU Study (2). There were advantages and disadvantages to this.

Advantages

It was clear from the OU Study (1) that the way in which care was given to dying residents was very dependent upon the registered manager's direction, since this was most often the person who developed procedures and practice in the home. Therefore any commitment to change would need to be initiated by the registered manager. For training to have an impact on policy and practice in the home it would have to be sanctioned by the registered manager. Beyond this their presence also signaled the importance of this area of training to the home staff.

Disadvantages

There were, however, disadvantages to their attendance and the tendency was for the registered manager to take a lead role in the workshop plenary sessions and some staff were inhibited by their presence. Not only was there a tendency for them to dominate the session but also, perhaps more worryingly, some registered managers presented an 'official line' on the practices within the home and defended aspects of care that could otherwise be deemed to be poor practice. In contrast, staff working in pairs and small subgroups were able to be more reflective and critical of the home's policy and practice and put forward their own ideas.

On balance the attendance of the registered manager at the training workshops had clear benefits. If participants are to be able to put their training into practice this will be dependent upon the support of the registered manager. The evidence from the nursing home palliative care training project (Smith 1998) is that, without the same level of awareness and knowledge shared by the registered manager, staff who tried to change their practice were unsuccessful and frustrated. The key to overcoming some of the disadvantages of registered manager attendance lies in good facilitation which is discussed later.

As well as the internal staff of the home we detected a need for training among some community nurses and some GPs. The GP was particularly important because the home staff were reliant on the GP to prescribe adequate pain relief to their residents.

The question of whether external support staff such as GPs and community nurses should take part in training alongside care home staff is one that the OU Study (2) investigated as part of the general issue of how training should take place in these settings.

External support involvement

Despite valiant attempts to encourage external professionals to attend the developmental training workshops in most homes there were no visiting staff present. The following is therefore based on a very small number of homes and is offered only as an impression. In the few workshops which they attended the experience also had advantages and disadvantages. It was an opportunity for home staff to benefit from their specialist knowledge in managing care. It was also a two way process in which external staff could appreciate the support home staff can offer when a resident is dying.

In some homes the community nurses, GPs, and Macmillan nurses who attended freely exchanged opinions with the care staff of the home. One GP who attended the focus group and then two subsequent workshops expressed a low degree of confidence in her palliative care skills. Her reason for attending the workshops was in part to learn from the carers' experiences which she valued highly. In another home a vigorous debate took place about the dying trajectories portrayed in the case studies and was continued in relation to home residents. In a large nursing home, the home physiotherapist and a care assistant challenged the GP's view about an ethical issue that had arisen in that home. Clearly this ability to discuss issues freely and also to learn from each other was a positive experience and one in which skills were shared. The presence of external staff was perhaps most useful in the workshop which dealt with pain and symptom management. The workshops raised the awareness of care staff to the need to evaluate pain and symptom treatment and the subsequent need to enlist the support of the GP attached to the home.

At the other end of the spectrum there was a tendency for the GP, community nurses and specialist palliative care nurses to dominate the groups and for the home staff to defer to them. In one home the staff deferred to the GP and left his views unchallenged. One key disadvantage in homes in which the views of the home staff were not equally valued was that the sharing of skills and knowledge appeared to be one-sided. The result was that there was not the same opportunity for care staff to demonstrate their skills. The success of the learning experience for the home staff was dependent upon recognizing and building on their skills.

Whatever are the merits of including GPs and other external staff in the training workshops in practice it is not likely that they will attend and so in reality the training will invariably be undertaken by internal staff only.

How to train?

Although lacking in formal training, staff in care homes have a lot of experience in dealing with death and dying. Many also have personal experience to draw on. Froggatt (2001) cautioned against education and training in palliative care which did not value the knowledge and experience already held by care staff. It was therefore a primary concern in designing the training materials for OU Study (2) that the knowledge and experience that staff already had should be central. In developing the training materials we took a learner-centred approach which moves away from the belief that an expert holds all the knowledge and skills and uses exercises and case studies to draw on all the participants' experience and understanding within a groupwork setting. This allows for different levels and abilities within the group to be accommodated.

Learner-centred learning groups can be defined as groups in which the following take place:

- the facilitator enables the experience, opinions, and knowledge of individual group members to be used as a basis for ideas, creativity, development, problem solving, and learning of the whole group
- everyone's experiences are treated as equally valuable and valid
- members share in the process of learning in the group, for example, by reflection, as well as engaging in the process of their own learning
- learning is active, participative and co-operative and is usually complementary to factual information which may be learned at a different time or delivered during the training session (e.g. lectures, demonstration or handouts) or
- learning is experiential, where new learning derives from reflection on activities which take place during a workshop or session (e.g. structured activities, case studies, role play).

(Adapted from Fletcher 1995)

The workshops, based on this type of group, were conducted in an experiential style and this was well received by staff who were not used to learning in this way. Case studies were used to avoid the need for personal disclosure and for people who had little experience of death and dying. Inevitably the workshops triggered feelings about loss in some participants and there were concerns about the ease with which people felt safe to disclose emotions that were thought to lie outside of the professional boundaries. Managing the emotional disclosures of staff is part of the skill of the group facilitator but throughout it is stressed that the workshops are learning not therapy groups. Whilst the group experience should be supportive certain boundaries have to be set at the outset which make the responsibility for disclosing personal emotional responses remain with the person making the disclosure. It is for them to seek help outside of the group.

Facilitation of the training workshops

The key to successful learner-centred learning groups which enable all participants within the group to feel valued lies in good facilitation. Participants need to feel safe to learn within a group setting and be encouraged to reflect on their practice. The facilitator therefore needs to be warm and friendly, encouraging, and not personally judgmental. Part of the teaching that is involved requires the facilitator to be able to use the ideas and the experiences that the participants bring to the workshops and turn them into teaching points. They need to value all the participants' contributions and experiences.

Managing the different levels of qualification and experience is something that requires a high level of skill on the part of the facilitator. Likewise, managing time and being responsive and flexible are important skills that are quite difficult to balance. Because this is so important we designed a set of training materials in OU Study (2) for the facilitator on how to run groups. This is supported by a video and gives guidance on group dynamics and models of group development, how to create and maintain a safe environment, how to set ground rules such as confidentiality and how to set objectives with the group. It also includes guidelines on how to promote participation within the group, to encourage active listening, to deal with emotional disclosures and to manage conflict.

Ideally we felt that an internal facilitator is preferable to someone from outside of the home. There is a danger that bringing in an outsider to facilitate the workshops perpetuates the belief that palliative care is not integral to the care of dying people in residential and nursing home settings. But this is a debatable point and we would also envisage that a Macmillan nurse or other specialist palliative care nurse or a community nurse could facilitate the workshops developed in OU Study (2) using the guidelines provided. How these materials were developed is addressed next.

The development of appropriate training materials

Having opted for a learner-centred approach within a groupwork setting which catered for all levels of staff it was important to provide within that framework training materials which met the needs of the participants. As a prelude to developing and testing training materials in OU Study (2) we used focus groups in homes to find out the type of training that staff themselves felt they needed. This enabled us to identify the areas of knowledge and expertise that staff felt they lacked.

High on the agenda of skills in need of further development was *communication* and in particular the skills required in talking to relatives of residents about death and dying. For example, some participants were concerned that they did not feel sufficiently confident to raise the subject of death and dying with residents and their relatives and when opportunities arose felt unable to respond adequately. The need for good *pain management* was considered to be an important element of caring for dying residents but many participants did not feel that they had adequate knowledge to manage this well, echoing the views of the Macmillan nurse expressed above. Not only did people request training in understanding about how to give analgesics effectively, but they also expressed the need for skills that would help them to liaise with GPs for better pain management. An understanding of how to control pain was part of the ability to negotiate more effectively. In some of the case study discussions, participants disclosed a reluctance to assess resident's pain because they felt powerless to respond. Also some participants were concerned about their ability to assess the pain of non-communicating residents.

Many participants expressed the need for training in *bereavement* care of families and to a lesser extent surviving residents. There were obvious tensions about whose responsibility it was to talk to families and some managers expressed concerns about carers who might assume the right to exceed their role following training but bereavement care and support was high on the list of training needs. The content areas which emerged and which were designed for testing were communication, pain and symptom management, bereavement care and support, ethical and cultural issues with an introductory workshop on the palliative care approach.

At the testing phase the most problematic of all the workshops was the workshop on *ethics*. This more abstract area had the greatest tendency to cause confusion among the participants. It was difficult for people to differentiate between the dimensions of practice, personal beliefs, and the law. Separating out *cultural issues* into one workshop topic also proved problematic as it naturally permeated all the other topics. It was decided therefore to integrate both ethical and cultural issues into all the other topics.

The final set of training materials developed consists of four free standing modules. A Foundation Module which provides an introduction to the palliative care approach, a Communication Module, a Pain and Symptom Management Module, and Bereavement Care Module. Each Module is made up of three workshops sessions. After carrying out the Foundation Module, the modules can be used in homes on a 'pick and mix' basis depending on their specific needs and preferences although we would recommend that they be used in the sequence listed above (Macmillan Cancer Relief, forthcoming).

Training levels

We were concerned about the level of the materials designed for workshops that would be attended by people with a mixture of skills and experience. The following three levels have been the guiding principles under which the training materials were developed.

The first level of raising awareness enables participants to recognize the needs of dying residents and their carers and is driven by activities that help participants to draw on their experience and to challenge thinking that is not based on evidence of good practice. The second level of knowledge and skills gives participants the evidence and skills they require in order to know how to respond to the needs of dying residents and their carers. It is not enough to know how to respond, however and participants need to understand how to put this knowledge and skills into practice. The third level enables participants to do this and therefore much of the workshop material in this area is based on role-play and simulation around case study material.

The format of the workshops

Each workshop has a set of aims and objectives which covers the basic know-ledge of the subject matter of each topic and the understanding and skills required to practice within the topic area. Each workshop begins with an introduction, where the programme of the session is introduced, the aims and objectives are reviewed and the ground rules set or confirmed. After the intro-duction the sessions are structured around different types of activities. Some take the form of general information/discussion activitiy where the facilitator leads a brainstorming activity or a discussion and inputs material in the form of handouts. Sometimes the whole group will be asked to break into small groups or to work in pairs where participants share aspects of personal or professional experiences or work on a set task such as a case study. This will usually be followed by a general feedback session where participants receive feedback from their small groups or pairs. Role play sessions are sometimes used to enable the participants to engage with issues experientially. Each workshop ends with a closing session where the workshop is reviewed and important points drawn out as well as sign posting the next workshop.

The workshops are structured into timed sessions with detailed guidance for the facilitator on how to run each session. Each one has a collection of sup-porting materials which include handouts, case studies, role play scenarios as well as audio materials. A set of readings is provided for the facilitator which give the background knowledge and understanding needed to run the session as well as a guide on how to run groups for those who may not have a great deal of experience.

Creating an environment for training

The experience of OU Study (2) clearly indicated that in order for training to be effective and to flourish there are certain conditions outside of the actual training materials which need to be addressed. Some are of a practical nature and relate to the context in which they are used while others have wider resource implications.

The context in which training takes place

Some of the more practical concerns that were raised in OU Study (2) had an important impact upon the quality of the learning experience. It was clear early on in the project that workshops were much more likely to be well received, well organized and also well attended in homes in which a training culture existed. Such a culture of training with a strong ethos of learning already existed in some homes involved in OU Study (2). These were usually nursing homes which had to fulfil their statutory requirement for trained nurses to keep their practice up to date. Where this was the case there also existed a tradition of teaching with non-trained staff, mainly within the NVQ structure.

The home as a training setting

The settings in which the training workshops took place were clearly limited by the home building and design but the rooms made available were an indication of the commitment made to training within the home. Certainly there was a clear correlation between homes in which training was seen as an important part of staff development and the facilities in which that development took place. A few homes had a training room and equipment which made for a more conducive environment. Staff were less likely to be interrupted in separate designated training areas. Where no such designated spaces were available some homes converted the staff room into a training space which ensured peace and quiet thus making training a priority for home staff.

In other homes it was difficult to find a space that was sufficiently separate from the main activities of the home and avoid the distractions and interruptions of the homes' daily routine and activities. In some homes the dining room was used and residents frequently strayed into the room and were ushered out by the staff. Using an area that residents shared and being visible to colleagues and visitors to the home made interruptions more likely to occur and was a serious distraction for participants. Although a training room set aside from the home's activities had clear advantages the room size also affected the participants' ability to take part in smaller group activities and role plays. Where homes are too small to provide adequate training facilities, the possibility could be explored of joining together with other homes in the vicinity to carry out the training.

The availability of staff to attend workshops

There is a major issue of staff being released from duties to attend the workshops. The experience from OU Study (2) when testing and piloting training materials was that staff were not always being released from their duties to attend the workshops and so were constantly being called away. There were homes in which 'on duty' staff attended the training workshop but were not 'on call', having been given cover by other members of staff. In a large number of the homes some of the participants attended in their own time, and a few of these were financially reimbursed or given time in lieu, but this was unusual. Problems arose when staff were either expected to attend in their own time or were on duty and likely to be called away to attend to duties in the home, such as taking a resident to the toilet or giving out the afternoon teas. In one example, some staff were called away up to five times during the session and in one extreme case in another home four of the five staff members left the workshop making it impossible to continue. There were also occasions when staff left the workshops at the time that they were meant to go off duty. Clearly this was highly unsatisfactory not only for themselves but also for the other group members who were left behind.

Continuity of participants is also important at the workshop sessions. Because staff bring different levels of knowledge and experience to their learning and because the workshops aim to build on that knowledge and understanding, if the group is to progress it is important that the composition of the group should not be constantly changing. In many homes where we ran more than one workshop topic different staff members attended different workshop topics. Consequently participants had to adapt to working with different group members and newcomers had to adjust to the highly interactive style of the workshops. It also meant that we could not assume that all participants had reached a level of knowledge and understanding from the previous session and so we had to repeat key areas of learning. Changing training group profiles makes it difficult for newcomers to understand and build upon knowledge from previous workshops.

Length of the workshops

Initially the workshops were intended to run for three hours but this was found to be impractical in many cases. Many of the problems of staff arriving late and leaving early, not being freed to attend the workshop would be eased if they were not so long. Also the ability of people to concentrate for long periods of time especially when they are not used to training situations was clearly an issue. It was therefore decided to hold shorter workshops of one and a half hours which gave people time to settle to the learning tasks and still hold useful discussions.

Wider resource implications

There are two major barriers to the widespread take up of training materials such as those developed in OU Study (2). The first is finance. It is unusual for homes to have a training budget and training tends to have a low priority. Local Authority and Voluntary homes were more likely to have a training budget but the majority of homes are privately run and they rarely have a budget for training. Where they do it is always vulnerable to a downturn in profits if home income is reduced by low resident occupancy.

The second is concerned with motivation and commitment. Carers do not necessarily find intrinsic value in training. They need to be motivated beyond its impact on their ability to deliver good quality care. This is not surprising in a workforce which is largely undervalued and underpaid. Carers need to be able to see the value of training in a meaningful way. This might be represented in some kind of tangible reward. There is a core of staff who see no need for training and the ability to overcome these barriers of resistance is a serious consideration.

Conclusion

Government documents (DoH 1999, 2001) have focused on the need for change in residential and nursing homes. Standards have been set for care in homes (DoH 2001). Standard 11 sets standards for caring for dying people. It is argued here that a key aspect in achieving this standard is training. We would thoroughly endorse the TOPSS (1999) proposal that this should be resourced as 'a tri-partite approach between employers, employees, and government to fund the necessary training to fill the knowledge, skills, and qualifications gap'. Without such a commitment, training will remain an activity undertaken only by homes already committed to improving care.

References

Counsel and Care. (1995) *Last Rites.* Counsel and Care, London.

Dalley, G. and Dennis, M. (2001) *Trained to Care? Investigating the Skills and Competencies of Care Assistants in Home for Older People.* Centre for Policy on Ageing Report No. 28. Centre for Policy on Ageing, London.

Department of Health. (1999) *Fit for The Future, Consultative Report.* Department of Health HMSO, London.

Department of Health. (2001) *Care Homes for Older People. National Minimum Standards.* Care Standards Act 2000. The Stationery Office, Norwich.

Fletcher, A. (1995) 'Learning in groups', in K502 *People and Potential.* The Open University.

Froggatt, K. (2000) *Palliative Care Education in Nursing Homes.* Macmillan Cancer Relief, London.

Froggatt, K. (2001) Palliative care and nursing homes: Where next? *Palliative Medicine,* 15, 42–8.

Katz, J.T., Sidell, M., and Komaromy, C. (2000) *Investigating the Training Needs in Palliative Care.* Unpublished report for the Department of Health.

Office for National Statistics. (1999) *Annual Abstract of Statistics.* The Stationery Office, London.

Shemmings, Y. (1996) *Death and Dying in Residential Care*. Avebury, Aldershot.

Sidell, M., Katz, J., and Komaromy, C. (1997) *Death and Dying in Residential and Nursing Homes For Older People: Examining the Case for Palliative Care*. Final Report to the Department of Health.

Smith, P. (1998) For the Palliative Care Education Pilot Project. *Report to the Steering Committee*, 22nd May 1998.

The Open University. (2002) *Death and Dying*, K260.

TOPSS, England. (1999) *Modernising the Social Care Workforce: The First National Training Strategy for England*. TOPSS, Leeds.

Chapter 9

Practical applications of the principles and practices of palliative care to the residential sector

Jeanne Katz

Assuming that it may be possible or even desirable to apply the elements of a philosophy which developed in setting one to another, this transference is fraught with difficulties. These can easily arise because of an arrogance that the first philosophy is in some ways superior and therefore should supplant the ethos or philosophy in the setting into which it is going to be transferred. The obvious conclusion is therefore that the second setting is wanting in some ways. However, the approbation of the hospice movement in recent years is not universal. Critiques cite, for example, the ways in which the hospice resembles some of the less desirable components of more conventional health care settings (e.g. institutionalization in James and Field 1992) or that hospices are more and more likely to only admit the most problematic cases, such as people with festering tumours (e.g. Lawton 1998). These suggest that the holy grail image of the hospice is already tarnished. And in any case why transplant a philosophy that is successful for a particular 'client group' to another. As Maddocks and Parker (2001) point out, nursing home residents may have different needs from hospice patients. Many of the former suffer from dementia and a lower proportion from cancer. This would suggest that 'palliative care providers should be cautious in assuming that knowledge and skills accrued in providing care for those dying from cancer can be directly transposed to the care of elderly people dying in nursing homes' (p. 149b). This chapter examines the transference of those skills.

As earlier chapters have indicated, staff in care homes in the first OU Study were quite determined that, where possible, dying residents should remain in their 'own homes' to die. The view that dying in one's own home is preferable to dying in an unfamiliar 'clinical' environment was widespread and echoes the views of the population in the United Kingdom (Townsend *et al.* 1990). As noted in Chapter 3, however, keeping dying residents in the home has a variety of implications for all concerned. And putting into practice the central tenet of palliative care, that is of enabling the dying person to exercise choice and control depends not only on the availability and perspectives of professional carers but also on the capability and capacities of the dying person him or herself.

Through the use of two case studies this chapter will identify the strengths of the palliative approach and opportunities for adapting this to people dying in residential care. The skills in question include a holistic approach, elements of communication skills, issues in relation to pain control as well as indicators about addressing the bereavement needs of all involved. Applying these may not only provide better care for dying residents in these settings, but also equip carers with a set of transferable skills, which should boost their confidence in caring for all residents with healthcare needs.

There are two important issues to bear in mind when reading the case studies given below: total pain, and whole patient care. The importance of maintaining the dying person's dignity is central to this chapter as indeed it is to the whole book.

Chapter 2 noted that there is currently more accommodation in residential homes than in nursing homes in the United Kingdom. For this reason this setting is the site for these case studies. 'Everglades Care Home' was chosen as it demonstrated good practice (relative to other homes studied in OU Study (1)). Chapter 10 will explore exclusively dying in nursing homes, albeit in the United States.

The first case study concerns 'Jack Perry' a resident who died of liver cancer. This illustrates some of the ways in which palliative care principles were applied to Jack's care, particularly early definitions of dying, but it also identifies some aspects of care that were lacking.

The second case study describes 'Margaret Scott', a lady with dementia who also died several weeks later in the same home following a number of transient ischaemic attacks. Her decline and death exemplifies points noted in Chapter 3 in relation to the dying trajectory of older people. Although Margaret had been ill for some time, the home staff were only certain that she was dying a few hours before her death. It proved to be difficult to provide pain relief in time to avoid Margaret becoming distressed: the researcher was able to observe the frustration of the home staff when they were unable to address Margaret's discomfort.

Background information about the home

Everglades Care home is a 32-bedded privately owned *residential* home in a seaside town in the South of England. Two ground floor wings with single en suite rooms lead off the main communal area which was the centre of the original house, and still accommodates 12 residents.

The staff

Although the owners do not manage the home, they are on site most days and play a role both in maintaining the fabric of the building and in relating to residents and their families and in particular liaise with social services about admissions. However, the day to day management is undertaken by the manager, Fiona Palmer, who works weekdays; she assesses residents and communicates with relatives, doctors, hospitals, and manages the day to day running of the home. She has two deputies, Hilary and Sandra. All of them have worked in Everglades for over eight years and they manage all day shifts and some night shifts. The large complement of staff from senior carers to kitchen staff are all long serving. Unusually for residential homes, staff turnover is minimal, even amongst the school girls who continue to work during holidays. There are several 'families' of staff represented with mothers, daughters, and sisters all part of the team.

Atmosphere in the home

It is a very friendly environment where staff joke and chat to residents but work extremely hard. The period during which the fieldwork took place was one of little change in the home despite the fact that many other homes had lost many residents over that Christmas period. Two years previously 11 residents had died over 12 months; the staff recalled this period with great distress.

Communication between staff members

Note taking is the central mechanism through which information is transmitted in Everglades. Before commencing a shift each care worker is required to read both the daily diary and a report book in which the leader of each shift notes important information about the residents. This includes social and practical information as well as 'nursing' issues. In addition, there is an individual book for each resident completed each day by the key worker but is not required reading for incoming staff, except where indicated in the report book. Any resident confined to bed has a care plan in the room which is completed each time staff members attend the resident. The systems therefore ensure that appropriate information is carefully conveyed to those who require it.

The residents

The residents are all white British local people, who have moved into Everglades from their own homes. Some residents are self-funding till their money runs out (Jack was an example of this), others are funded by the local authority. The home always has a waiting list. Most residents are ambulant and participate in some of the many activities laid on for them by the staff and outside people. The residents are extremely happy in the home:

> But here it is such a peaceful place. So utterly peaceful.

During the study period most residents were self-caring and aware of what was happening in the home. They felt able and keen to communicate with the researcher about almost any issue.

Relationship with visitors

The home was always very busy with visitors, district nurses, chiropodists, and hairdressers. Relatives were seen to be an integral part of residents' care and often took them out. Where there were no relatives, the staff ensured that residents who wished to go out, could and did. Relatives were kept in close touch with the medical status of the residents and were called when someone was ill and expected to participate in decision making. Relatives were encouraged to participate in the care.

Caring for dying residents

Everglades care home has a policy document regarding procedures in case of death. (This conforms with 11.12 National Minimum Standards for Care Homes, see Chapter 2.) This is framed in the office for all to see. It makes explicit the following philosophy:

> At Everglades we like to give residents peace of mind that this is their home until death, and they do not have to worry at the first sign of a physical/mental problem they'll be moved elsewhere. Wherever possible we will care for them in every way possible, using the support of GPs, nursing services, and of course, the family.
>
> When death is imminent this care will be in the resident's own room and as dignified as possible.
>
> (See full policy in appendix at the end of this chapter.)

The philosophy is to keep residents requiring basic nursing care in the home as long as possible, but sometimes the nursing requirements become too complex to manage. For example, during fieldwork there was concern about how the district nurse was caring for a resident with a supra-pubic catheter. Fiona was sent on a course to learn how to manage it. However this eventually became too complicated and the resident was transferred to a *nursing* home.

Staff training in the home was done primarily in-house and most of the carers were registered for NVQs. As noted above, occasionally senior carers were sent on external courses to learn specific skills. However, none of the carers had received any training in relation to palliative or bereavement care despite day sessions being available at the local hospice.

Staff of all grades maintained that wherever possible residents should die in their own beds and attempted to provide the appropriate emotional and nursing care themselves. The range of nursing care was limited. Nevertheless two previous residents had been fitted with syringe drivers. Syringe drivers had not been an unqualified success in the home: carers expressed concern with the amount of medication prescribed and suggested that some residents were dying in unnecessary pain. Additionally they questioned the competence of the district nurses responsible for overseeing the management of the syringe drivers. (However, none of the carers had received specific training in managing syringe drivers, nor indeed in the principles of pain relief.) Despite the fact that there was a hospice nearby and three Macmillan nurses in the area, on no occasion had they been contacted for advice: the district nurse and GP had taken responsibility for the care of the syringe driver.

The account of how Jack's illness was managed is constructed primarily from his case notes which chronicle Jack's entire stay in Everglades. These were kept in the office and were the main documented form of communication between staff in the home. In addition to these case notes, other perspectives about his care were gathered through interviews with his sister Ann, his GP Dr Fraser, Fiona Palmer the home manager, and other members of the care home staff. The origin of all the quotes are identified but to preserve anonymity the names have been changed. The researcher was not in the home when Jack died.

The management of Jack Perry's illness

Jack Perry was a 76-year old divorcé who prior to his admission to Everglades lived nearby in his own flat. He was in close touch with both his sisters but had complicated relationships with his ex-wife, his son and two daughters all of whom lived locally. Jack's sister Ann corroborated Dr Fraser's explanation for Jack's admission to Everglades Residential Home 'a sort of family social services style admission, because of a deteriorating ability to cope on his own at home. And it was actually just round the corner from where he lived'. Ann recalled that Jack had been admitted a year previously for a short stay following surgery for cancer. His admission summary noted that Jack had a physical disability, and suffered from glaucoma 'for which he needs eye drops'. It continued:

> Although Mr Perry coped for a while on his return home, it would appear that the cancer is not under control completely and he continues to require radiotherapy so he has decided to move into Everglades permanently.

Home manager Fiona Palmer recalled Jack's previous admission:

> Jack came to us originally as a short stay following surgery. He had a sigmoid colectomy because they discovered he'd got cancer of the colon, and they had actually cleared it completely. And he was quite frail, and so he came to us initially for a short time. And then he found that he couldn't cope living at home. And he came in to us and unfortunately he gradually developed cancer of the liver.

She summed up Jack's care and in particular the relationship with Dr Fraser as follows:

> And the doctor that saw him was absolutely brilliant with him. He'd actually diagnosed without xray that he'd got a recurrence of cancer. But he didn't tell him. He said: Let me know when he's ready and, you know, I will tell him. And, although Jack was convinced that he'd got cancer, he thought he'd got lung cancer . . . And eventually, when he was very poorly, Dr Fraser said to him: You know what's wrong. And Jack said: Yes I've got lung cancer. And he said: No actually you haven't, you've got—and he apparently didn't want to discuss it, because he was convinced that he'd got lung cancer, and that he was going to have a horrific death, like haemorrhaging and that. And he was frightened of how it would affect him, and how it would affect us and how it would affect his family. And, when he was told that it was not that, he kind of relaxed a bit I suppose. The surgery were very supportive of him. The family wanted him to stay here. He was given the choice if he wanted to stay—and he didn't want to go anywhere else. And he died peacefully here really. You know, they set up all the equipment for him. He had intravenous morphine and everything. The surgery was very supportive.

According to Dr Fraser, Jack's underlying and most central 'medical issue' was:

> He had colon cancer with quite significant liver involvement. [People in this situation] seem to do fairly well for a while and then deteriorate quite rapidly. And that's what happened with him really. It was probably no more than six weeks before his death he started to deteriorate quite significantly, with more pain, and less mobility, and less intake of food.

Jack deteriorates

Jack's case notes tell the story as it happened. The following excerpts highlight some of the main care issues. Three weeks after Jack's admission it was noted that:

> He is settling down more now, it has been quite difficult for him, more so than he expected. He is experiencing considerable pain in his shoulder which he is spraying with Ralgex as the cream that was being rubbed in in the evenings was not having much effect.

Throughout all the accounts, Jack's shoulder and arm pain continue to plague him as his main site of discomfort. With hindsight Dr Fraser acknowledged that the urgent reason for his admission was

> . . . an unrelated problem which was his main obsession, a pain in his arms and legs, which I don't think we ever really sorted out what that was due to. And I still think to this day it was probably more related to an arthritic process than anything else. But of course as his general physical condition deteriorated, then the pain in his shoulder became more of a problem. . .

The shoulder pain was addressed initially and then subsequently by cortisone injections administered at the surgery but gave Jack little relief. Although many efforts were made by the home and the primary care team to address this pain pharmacologically or through other means, this remained Jack's main source of aggravation and pain.

Two weeks after Jack's admission to Everglades his case notes report:

> Visited by his sister this afternoon. Sadly their sister passed away unexpectedly yesterday. Apparently Jack was very close to her and will be absolutely devastated. We will support him as much as possible. Given a tray of tea to have with his family.

The care staff at Everglades were sensitive to the bereavements experienced not only by relatives of deceased residents and staff themselves but also to the fact that residents may themselves be bereaved outside of the home and need supporting. This quote suggests that support would be offered and the practical response was to ensure that the family could drink tea together.

Jack was taken by the home owner to the local hospital for a planned colonoscopy which was preceded by his need to take medication to empty his bowels prior to this. The case notes emphasized his 'nil by mouth' and 'instructions left out for staff to follow'.

Over the subsequent few weeks, his case notes repeatedly focused on unsuccessful attempts by the surgery to address Jack's shoulder pain including changes of medication. *There is no suggestion here that a specialist palliative care nurse should be consulted, or that Jack should be referred to a pain clinic.* The case notes note the extent of Jack's pain and occasional visits to the surgery and a private physiotherapist and Jack's decision to acquire a TENS machine. However, his discomfort levels are so acute that the case notes record on 7 January:

> Fiona Palmer (home manager) extremely concerned about the amount of pain Jack is in and his general deterioration as its consequence. Jack is not eating very

well at the moment and is having very disturbed nights, plus is taking an awful amount of painkillers with little result. Dr Fraser contacted for home visit.

Dr Fraser attended 12 noon. Although in no doubt that Jack has a shoulder problem of long standing Dr more concerned that general deterioration may be due to secondary cancer of liver this time. Is going to arrange for a scan at local hospital asap but for obvious reasons has said nothing of his suspicions to Jack. Dr Fraser is happy to talk to Jack's children either before or after scan depending on whether they ask us for any details. Should the scan confirm Dr Fraser's suspicions then the course of treatment will probably be pain control only (details of pain killers noted—to continue taking diclofenac, Dr Fraser suggested Jack take both at same time. MST may make Jack sleepy at first, this is normal).

The following few weeks' case reports detail Jack's slow deterioration—a growing concern that his pain has not receded, but a general impression is gained that Jack is managing better emotionally. His younger daughter had phoned to enquire how the next scan had gone, and had visited him the following day.

Two weeks later the case notes illustrate how the GP altered Jack's drugs and also his attitude towards discussing Jack's illness with him:

21st January
    Visited by Dr Fraser. Has altered Jack's medication as follows:
    [Details of drugs] . . . will hopefully restore Jack's appetite but does not always work. However it will always help Jack's chest.
    Jack did not actually ask Dr Fraser what the scan shows so Dr Fraser has not told him, he prefers to wait for the patient to ask.
    The scan has shown that there is now 'activity' in this area which is untreatable and Dr Fraser is of the opinion that Jack's shoulder pain could also be caused through a similar 'activity'. Dr Fraser does not feel that Jack will benefit from investigations to the shoulder considering his liver condition. Dr aims to keep Jack as comfortable as possible.
    Jack is aware that there is more to the scan than just his shoulder—he is of the opinion that the cancer—'it' as Jack refers to it, is all over his body. I have explained to Jack that Dr Fraser is quite willing to come in to see him and answer questions when Jack is ready. Jack is going to wait until he has seen his children—who he knows have had contact with Dr Fraser.

A few days later (25 January) the case notes report that *Jack is struggling a bit today. . . Doubling the MST will hopefully ease his discomfort; we are doing all we can to help Jack cope and be as comfortable as possible*. This pattern continued for some days until the first mention of what must have been a recurrent additional symptomatic problem: *Still complaining of constipation. I spoke with Dr Fraser who has advised 2 × Senna at night and to continue with the rest of medication. He will see Jack next week.*

The following entry demonstrates the careful balance between facilitating dying people to manage their medication and the science of pain control:

> A reasonable week for Jack, he has his good and bad days. He is suffering considerable pain as the MST wears off. Last night he wanted to leave his pills until late, but Hilary (senior carer on duty) explained the importance of taking his medication at regular times.

A week later (2 February), the entry demonstrates a deterioration in Jack's condition:

> Jack is looking very tired and frail most of the time now. His appetite comes and goes in waves, if all else fails he enjoys a cheese and pickle sandwich. Everyone supports as much as possible, and Jack regularly thanks us for this.

This deterioration is marked by some 'general health' observations, such as a decision not to give Jack a flu injection, and noting that Jack now was experiencing diarrhoea and nausea. Doctor was visiting several times per week and increased the MST. One note useful for others reading the case notes concerned the effect the MST may have on Jack:

> This increase may make Jack feel 'whoosy' for a couple of days but to persevere with it.

Dr Fraser noted that Jack's liver feels considerably enlarged compared to an examination seven days previously.

The following day (3 February) is the turning point in Jack's deterioration as staff at Everglades embarked on a care plan. This would suggest that the care staff in conjunction with the GP have defined Jack as dying. For only the third time, a syringe pump is going to be set up in the home. There is no suggestion that the palliative care physician or the hospice team might visit to support the staff. At the same time, there is no indication that at any time, the team feel anything other than confident and competent to manage Jack in the home till his death.

The case notes read as follows:

> Jack deteriorating quite rapidly, in severe pain, finding it difficult to take medication, unable to drink very much. Contacted Dr Fraser.
>
> a.m. Care plan started. Seen by Dr Fraser who discussed his condition with him. Jack knew he had cancer but thought it was in the lungs. Dr Fraser told him that it was in the liver. Dr Fraser is arranging for district nurse to call and fit morphine pump and has explained how it works to him. District nurse will then call in daily to check him.
>
> p.m. District nurse Tom called to fit syringe drive pump. Will call regularly every 24 hours to check pump. Jack became anxious over pump—visited by

daughters who seem to disturb him quite a lot. Unable to eat anything at the moment, but drinking.

Nearing death

For the next week until Jack's death eight days later, there were daily entries in the case notes. Jack was checked by the district nurse and was visited by his family, but was rather unsettled and disturbed the pump. On the 9 February, Dr Kennedy, another doctor from the surgery, who knew Jack well, visited and placed the needle in another site. The following day (10 February) Jack was still in considerable pain and Dr Kennedy agreed by phone to increase the morphine. At this point either Dr Fraser or Dr Kennedy were coming in each day; additionally all Jack's children visited but according to the case notes, *'Jack tends to become agitated and restless when they are around'*. The notes indicate that Jack was very thirsty and drinking a lot, still not sleeping and in pain. Dr Fraser visited and prescribed temazepam to help Jack sleep but this was not effective and Jack had a disturbed night and was in considerable pain the following morning:

> (11th February) Dr Fraser contacted for diamorphine increase—to 400 mg per 24 hours, cyclizine increased to 100 mg per 24 hours. D/nurse expected this to make Jack quite drowsy. However, no real effect on Jack until later in the evening.

The next day was a better one for Jack, insofar as he had slept a bit during the night. He was much calmer although not eating and incontinent. As the two doctors familiar with Jack were off duty a third doctor from the surgery (Dr Needham) attended and 'was satisfied' and decided not to alter Jack's medication. The case notes for the 12 February noted administering temazepam to Jack at 10 p.m., and that he appeared 'calm with laboured breathing'. Also he was *'checked regularly throughout the night; marked deterioration in his condition, and that his breathing became shallow and bubbly'*. What could be noted here, is that it was apparent that Jack was now approaching death, but there is no suggestion that he would want or require someone to sit with him throughout the night. However at 4 a.m., it was noted that the *'battery in syringe driver replaced with one from the shop as flashing on machine had stopped'*.

In the morning (13 February) the syringe driver was still playing up and the duty doctor contacted at 7 a.m. for assistance. Twenty minutes later Dr Needham, who had seen Jack the previous day returned the call:

> 6.45 We explained that we had had problems with syringe driver since 4.20 am and have had to manually dose Jack on and off since 5 am. Dr confirmed that we would not be overdosing Jack by continuing manually and to contact

the surgery at 8.30 for district nurse to come and sort out pump. Manually dosing at approx. 15 minutes intervals if not showing flashing light on driver.

Manager tried to get through to surgery till 8.45 before she went off duty. 8.45 I (carer in charge) eventually got through to surgery, explained the situation. District nurse is being bleeped for an immediate visit.

9.15 District Nurse, Susan Butters, visited, feels it was the battery at fault, new one fitted. She also completely changed tubing and resited (the needle) on top of left arm as no flesh left on chest. Driver appears to be working well now but Susan will arrange for a twilight nurse to come in and check all is working correctly.

Jack given gentle wash and change of pyjama top, also creamed all pressure areas. Jack as comfortable as possible. Conveen fitted, no drainage in bag as only mouth wash now. Visited by daughter Julie for a little while shortly afterwards. Jack's breathing becoming increasingly laboured. Fingers started to blue up more as morning progressed.

11.45 Jack twitching and moving about quite a bit so contacted district nurse re increase of morphine.

12.0 Jack visited by his sister Ann and brother-in-law Dave. I explained that I didn't think it would be long now and that we were awaiting the district nurse to call and increase the morphine. They said they would sit with him.

12.05 Susan phoned to say that Dr Needham had agreed to increase the morphine.

12.15 Susan arrived. Jack passed peacefully away as we walked into the room. Ann was with him. District Nurse contacted Dr Needham. I requested her to remove pump which she did.

12.45 Dr Needham called to confirm (death). Telephoned the oldest child who said she would contact all the family herself. Wasn't sure whether burial or cremation. Later rang to confirm cremation. Funeral directors contacted and will call to collect Jack's body at 2 pm.

2. 00 watch, rings and small change put in envelope in file.

Discussion

Jack's care raises a number of important issues for end-of-life care many of which will be picked up at the end of the chapter. Jack was one of a sizeable minority of residents, but a minority nevertheless, who died of cancer with concomitant pain. Until the last week of his life, the discomfort that bothered him the most had possibly nothing to do with the malignancy, his shoulder and arm pain, and although he attended the surgery frequently, this pain was never stemmed. At no time did the three doctors who attended him suggest that he attend a pain clinic, nor was a pain physician consulted. The syringe driver was set up in the home by the District Nurse but there were several difficulties with this. This included a perception that Jack's pain was never properly addressed. The home staff were not entirely comfortable with the competence of either the pump itself nor the nurses supervising it; all the carers might have benefited from a visit from the specialist palliative care team which served the area. In relation to communication, the carers were very clear that the most appropriate person to discuss Jack's illness with him was the doctor. The staff did not attempt to talk to him about this, nor about his relationships with his family, whose visits clearly distressed him and possibly aggravated his pain.

In contrast to Jack, Margaret Scott's illness and demise was more typical of a care home resident. She suffered from multi-infarct dementia and this had progressed to the point where she hardly communicated. The beginning of her dying phase was less easy to pinpoint than Jack's.

The death of Margaret Scott

Margaret (known as Maggie) Scott died when the researcher was present in Everglades. This account is reconstructed from the researcher's notes, the case notes, the care plan and interviews with Maggie's doctor, Dr Reynolds, and several members of the home staff. (Maggie was registered with a different surgery to Jack.)

Maggie was an 87-year-old woman who had been admitted to Everglades eight months previously because she was no longer coping in her own environment. The staff described her condition as stroke-induced dementia. Maggie's speech has been affected as she had dysphasia. At first the staff felt that she knew what she wanted to say, but the words were not coming out right. Ten days before she died Margaret seemed to have had an attack of some kind. The case notes read as follows:

> Maggie appears to have had an episode of some sort. 11 am, bed absolutely saturated. It's thought she had suddenly let go. Maggie unresponsive, unable to stand or co-ordinate, not even open her eyes. Dr Reynolds contacted. Maggie given bed wash and complete change of bedding and night wear. Unable to take drink, mumbling words, not making any sense, settled back into bed.
>
> Seen by Dr Reynolds, feels she's had a TIA (transient ischaemic attack), and possibly a mini-stroke also. Doesn't want to attempt any radical treatment. Advises we keep her comfortable. She may recover from this, but he's hopeful that nature will take its course, especially in view of her quality of life now. Maggie dry and comfortable. If she appears to feel any pain he will prescribe MST. Doesn't want us to call out another doctor out of hours as he doesn't feel anything will be gained by hospital admission, unless we are unable to manage. Dr Reynolds is on duty tonight himself, so he may very well call in himself to check her. Dr Reynolds has spoken to her son Tim at length, explained the situation fully. Tim is in complete agreement. Tim will be contacting Margaret's brother, and sister, who may very well visit. Tim would like to be informed of any drastic changes, and will visit himself in the next couple of days.

The GP, Dr Reynolds, corroborated the home's version of the incident. He decided to keep Margaret in Everglades because:

> There had been a step wise deterioration in Margaret's condition over the past few months. Two weeks ago she had a fairly large event and we'd already discussed things in the past, to wait a bit and see if she came round. I went to see her, she'd lost her gag reflex which is something new which would mean that she couldn't swallow, a fairly terminal event, prognostically bad for strokes... I decided at this point not to admit her under my care (to the cottage hospital or the main hospital) because I felt confident in the competency in the home. I considered this, but decided against it because I felt the staff at the home would not panic. I discussed it with the son and said I would rather leave her there, he agreed. From that point she made an almost full recovery and coping well, back to square one. It was a bit of a shock, how well she did, actually...
>
> Two days before she died, it was already decided that it was tender loving care, terminal care. She was again given a certain amount of assessment to see whether she improved and when she failed to improve and was complaining of abdominal pain, that's when I decided to give her more active palliative care. I started off with oramorph because you can increase or decrease the dose; I don't think she ever got the suspension.

The doctor explained that in these circumstances he would not get a Macmillan nurse as the illness would be too short a duration. He would normally have involved district nurses, but again there were:

> certain places where I have confidence that where I give instructions they are passed on to the next person coming on—this is where I often feel homes fall down, it's fine for the person to whom I explain things—you then move down to the next person, and there's another phone call, summoned out at night and it all goes to pot.

The following day's entries read as follows:

> Maggie's plain band ring was becoming loose, removed for safety. Found on bedroom floor at 6.45 am. Helped back to bed. Washed and dressed later, brought down to lounge, but she's still very unsteady. Very sleepy, not very stable when walking. This evening unable to eat or drink anything.
>
> 4.2. Up and dressed and brought downstairs. Visited by family... became very white and closed her eyes. Wheelchaired to her room with some difficulty. Undressed and padded, possibly another CVA. Unable to take sips of liquid. Arms moving, but legs extremely weak. No medication able to be taken, but Margaret does not appear to be in any pain.
>
> 5.2. Found lying across bed without any covers on, muttering to herself. Magazines all over floor. Helped back to bed. Margaret refused to open her eyes.

The staff explained how they viewed what was going on:

> We weren't sure what it was, whether it was a TIA, or a mini-stroke. And she recovered from that, but she wasn't as well as she was before. And she's been quite frail really since. I think she . . . not eating very well, not drinking very well. But we had her up and dressed and brought her downstairs, and she was actually sitting down having—well, at the supper table, when suddenly, she just went as white as a sheet, closed her eyes—So the girls had to put her in her wheelchair and take her upstairs and put her into bed. And that's where she's been ever since. And she's been muttering, and mumbling.

The staff noticed that Margaret kept hugging her tummy. When the GP checked her stomach Margaret didn't react. The manager reported that the GP said:

> we'll just keep her comfortable, and I'll ring in the morning and see how she is. And he said, I think, you know, if she's still disturbed, we'll—if she hasn't made any recovery, then I'll start her on MST, to keep her comfortable.

The day she died

The following morning Margaret's breathing was reported as erratic and laboured. The staff commented that she did not appear conscious and the only time she responded was when they turned her. Although Dr Reynolds had left strict instructions that no other doctor should be called, he was off duty. Fiona hoped that his partner, Dr Long, whom she had called to see another resident might advise them on how best to handle the situation. The staff told the researcher that they were popping in every quarter of an hour or so to observe Margaret.

By lunch time the home staff were certain that Margaret was dying. They noted that her swallowing reflex had gone and that she seemed semi-conscious. Consequently they instituted changes in the layout of her room to facilitate nursing as well as a care plan to be filled out each time a member of staff went into her room. When pressed about how long it might take, the two senior members of staff estimated a few days, this being Thursday, probably over the weekend. The manager had already spoken to Margaret's son twice and intended to phone again after the doctor had been.

On entry into Margaret's room the changes made were evident. The care plan was sited on Margaret's dresser. It detailed all the observations at every visit to her room, plus descriptions of the pain relief efforts. Margaret's bed had been moved around so that it was possible to access Margaret from both sides. Normally the one side of the bed was against the wall, and therefore it was difficult to get round her.

Hilary, the deputy manager explained their philosophy of caring for a dying resident in Margaret's room. The key worker and/or a manager was popping in very regularly to see Margaret but their practice was not to sit with dying residents. Several reasons were given. One was that they did not have enough time available. A second was that staff become hypnotized by the breathing and then tended to go to sleep themselves. In addition, sitting with a dying person could be very distressing.

Physical care and emotional support of the dying person were priorities. The physical care included putting Vaseline on her lips frequently. There was a little swab next to Margaret's bed so that they could drip water into her mouth to try to prevent dryness. Margaret's pressure areas were checked regularly. At one point she was lying on her back, and she only had two pillows, although her breathing was extremely shallow and noisy. They had just taken away a third pillow, because it was very important to keep changing her position.

The senior staff and key worker were continuing to check on Margaret very frequently, one of them every ten or fifteen minutes. She was lying in bed and seemed to be semi-conscious. The staff had had difficulty with the MST solution which did not fit into the container supplied by the chemist for that purpose, so that they had to dissolve the solution within the syringe, which was completely impractical and rather difficult. They had tried unsuccessfully to drip the MST solution into her mouth with a syringe but this was unsuccessful because she seemed to have lost her swallowing reflex.

Whenever a staff member entered the room they communicated quietly with Margaret. They stroked her gently, and explained precisely what was happening, hoping to get some kind of response. Mary, the key worker, checked to see whether the arms or the legs were stiffening, and also pointed out to the researcher that Margaret's hands were going very blue. She thought that the end was not that far away.

Hilary emphasized that they explained to the dying person what they were doing, and why they were there. She believed that often the hearing remains even after someone has died, and therefore one had to be very cautious with what one said. Having said that, she kept talking about the fact that death was very imminent, in the room. So she was having two conversations, one with Margaret and one with the researcher, both equally loud.

The staff became progressively more anxious for the doctor to arrive and adjust the medication, because it clearly was not working. The reason given for the prescription of MST powder, although it wasn't clear that she was in pain, was that MST was a sedative, sometimes hastening death. In addition the staff felt that administering the MST would reduce Margaret's agitation.

On arrival Dr Long agreed that, as her swallowing reflex was not working, it would be a good idea for her to have MST suppositories (he rejected Fiona's suggestion of a syringe driver). However he had left his prescription pad behind and therefore somebody would have to collect the script from the surgery before going to the chemist. Fiona commented:

> Well, I was appalled. Because, I mean, our first consideration was the comfort of the resident. Fortunately Margaret wasn't in any discomfort. But we weren't prepared for her to die so quickly. We wanted to make sure she was comfortable while we were caring for her. I mean, the fact that I had to chase around was ridiculous really, wasn't it? I mean, if he'd have brought his prescription pad in, at quarter to three I'd have been up to the pharmacy, and she would have had (her medication immediately).

The staff noted no change in Margaret's condition. When the other deputy manager, Sandra, arrived she, Mary, the key worker and Fiona went upstairs to change Margaret's position and put her on her side. As there were only two care workers on the evening shift, they took the opportunity to turn Margaret when the new shift came on duty. She was a very tall and fairly heavy woman, and this explained the difficulty in changing her position.

Before Fiona left, she went to see Margaret again. There was a definite change in her condition—her legs were now going blue and her hands completely so. The staff were most anxious to get the MST suppositories as they felt Margaret might be in pain. However not only had the doctor come out without his prescription pad, he now discovered that the chemist would not take a prescription for MST by fax, therefore Fiona had to go and collect the prescription from the surgery. The tension was exacerbated by the fact that none of the town's chemists stocked this suppository so Fiona had to go to an adjacent town to collect the drugs. She finally returned with the suppositories at five to five to the relief of her staff.

Sandra, the deputy manager ran upstairs to administer the drugs and immediately the buzzer sounded with a great urgency. Margaret had died in the interim.

Contact with the family

Throughout the day the staff had been in touch with Margaret's son, Tim who had rung on the last occasion when Fiona had been at the chemist. Sandra had spoken to him and had said death was fairly imminent, and now, twenty minutes later, she had to ring back to tell him that Margaret had died. Normally she would have waited until the death had been certified, but she was very concerned that Tim was travelling from London, and he needed to know before he set out on his journey hoping to see his mother alive. Sandra decided not to phone Tim on the mobile, because the news of his mother's death would distress him so she therefore contacted his wife.

Having notified the son and the surgery, Sue and Brenda, the care assistants on duty, tidied Margaret. They did not lay her out. They felt that it's quite intrusive to the dying person, and that was the undertaker's role. They tried to make Margaret look comfortable.

The surgery phoned back to say that the duty doctor, Dr Long, would not be coming to certify Margaret's death, as he was perfectly sure that Sandra was capable of ascertaining that she was dead. Assuming that Margaret would be taken to the local funeral director, he said he'd pop into the mortuary at some point and check on her. Sandra was absolutely furious that he would not come and certify her death, noting that this was illegal. Fifteen minutes later there was a call from Margaret's son, Tim who told her that she should go ahead and organize for his mother to be taken to the funeral director. At 6 o'clock, Margaret's own doctor, Dr Reynolds, who had originally instructed that nobody else should be called, arrived. Although off duty, he was at the surgery when he overheard that Margaret had died, and decided to come himself to certify her death.

Dr Reynolds felt strongly about continuity of care and wanted to certify Margaret himself. In addition he wanted to collect the drugs and ensure that they were disposed of properly. He examined her, and wrote on the death certificate that she had died of: (1) Cerebral Vascular Accident, and (2) Multi-Infarct Dementia.

On Dr Reynolds's departure there were some further calls with the family. It was unclear whether either Tim or his mother's sister, who lived nearby, would visit. The carers needed this information as it had implications for removing Margaret's body. Sandra had asked the funeral directors to come during dinner time because that meant that all the residents would be in the dining room, and it would facilitate removing Margaret from the home. Because Margaret was large and lived on the first floor, she would have to have been brought down on a stretcher, in the lift. The funeral directors arrived at twenty past six, at the same time as Margaret's sister and brother-in-law. Sandra asked the funeral directors to wait in their hearse until Margaret's relatives had been upstairs to see her. Sandra noted that it was appropriate that they had not laid Margaret out because this meant that her sister saw Margaret in as natural a position as possible.

Once the family had left, the funeral directors went up to Margaret's room and the researcher was asked to ensure that residents did not leave the dining room. This created an interesting problem, because several of the residents were extremely keen to go out after their meal. The undertakers took some time to get Margaret onto the stretcher. To secure her they had to tie her with straps resembling seat belts, before placing her in the lift and taking her out.

Sandra said that she preferred residents to die on her shift, because it gave her an opportunity to say good-bye. She said:

> we're all very possessive round here, we all like the residents to die on our own shift, because we then feel that we have an opportunity to say good-bye and do the last thing for them.

Sandra accompanied the funeral directors to the hearse 'seeing' Margaret on her way. All but two of the surviving residents were still in the dining room. They were aware that Margaret was ill by her absence from dinner. Many intuitively had guessed that she had died by the urgency with which the bell had rung. They seemed unsettled but Sandra believed that it was wrong to tell people that somebody has died just before they go to bed, because they then dwelt on it. Residents were able to corroborate, explain and justify this method of communicating information. Most were told officially the following day by Fiona; despite being together when she died they had chosen not to discuss it till it was openly acknowledged.

However, two residents knew, a woman who had 'escaped' and passed the undertakers on the stairs and a blind resident who was already in her room listening very carefully:

> Sandra came through and said to me 'I'm going to close the door, Mrs Court'. And I thought, another one died. You see, they never close doors...and I thought well, somebody upstairs has been ill for about a week...

Once Margaret had been taken away, arrangements began to be made for her funeral. Her son had hoped that it would leave from the home:

> I said to Fiona, can we run the funeral from there, if I pay you. If a few people can come back, you know, and get your chef and we'll have a room there and we just have a cup of tea. Because I said, being as it was the last place she lived, I thought it would be nice to do it from there. She said, 'Look I'd like to, but we can't do anything like that. Because we don't let anyone you know. You can't have the funeral from the home. Too distressing for the other residents and all the rest of it'. And I said, 'oh yes, that's fair enough.'

Discussion

Margaret's death unsettled the staff at Everglades primarily because they felt impotent in ensuring that she had sufficient pain control. Although carers are untrained in assessing need for medication, those on duty during Margaret's last hours were distressed that Margaret may have died in pain and discomfort.

Understandings of palliative care

Palliative care encompasses basic human rights as well as focusing on the dignity and centrality of the dying person. The staff felt reasonably happy that they had enabled both Jack and Margaret to die in 'their own home' and exercise choice and control. In Margaret's case this was harder to demonstrate given her mental capabilities, but her son could be seen as a proxy. There is no doubt that in many other homes, both Jack and Margaret may have been admitted to hospital.

We now explore the care of Jack and Margaret within the context of both the principles of palliative care, and Standard 11 of the National Minimum Standards outlined in Chapter 2 (see p. 37–8). The outcome of this standard states: *Service users are assured that at the time of their death, staff will treat them and their family with care, sensitivity and respect.* [Where a practice exemplifies a substandard, the number of that substandard is appended, e.g. 11.x].

Predicting death

As noted in Chapters 3 and 4, predicting death for younger people with cancer is considerably easier than for older people with chronic degenerative conditions, such as heart failure or strokes. Care staff in encountering older people on a daily basis may not notice very gradual deterioration or even increase in pain. Most older people in care homes suffer from a variety of ailments, some of which compromise their quality of life or may be life-threatening but many they have 'learned to live with'. Recognizing early enough that someone may be in a downward spiral, regardless of whether they die at the predicted time, facilitates the process of organizing and providing appropriate care. Both Margaret and Jack were seen by staff as nearing death and predictions were made as health workers are wont to do using the temporal strategies identified by Glaser and Strauss (1968). However, in both cases if strategies for care, particularly in relation to pain control could have been put into place much earlier these might have avoided the unnecessary 'panics' at the end stages.

Enabling the dying person to retain control

Enabling the dying person to retain control is central to the palliative approach. Similarly, standard 11.9 of the National Minimum Standards states '*The changing needs of service users with deteriorating conditions or dementia—for personal support or technical aids—are reviewed and met swiftly to ensure the individual retains maximum control*'. Margaret was no longer able to express her wishes in relation to terminal care and arrangements after death (11.3) but Jack was clear that he wanted to remain in the home surrounded by his personal belongings (11.6).

Pain control and symptom relief

Regardless of whether the cause of pain is cancer, dementia, heart disease or kidney failure, people dying in all settings require good pain control and symptom relief. Skilled pain and symptom assessment is essential to ensure smooth management. This is not an easy task with older people who may be very frail and have multiple physical health problems confounded by difficulties in communicating. Despite the fact that more people aged 65 die of cancer than those under 65 (raw figures not percentages) older people in all settings do not seem to access palliative care services in the expected numbers (Addington Hall and Higginson 2001). Poor pain control in older people may in fact be a symptom of ageism, a view that older people are not seen as appropriate for palliative care (ibid.; OU Study (1)).

Carers in Everglades were not trained to be familiar with signs or symptoms of pain or distress in order to make a recommendation to physicians when to commence analgesia (see Chapter 8). Attempting to persuade physicians to introduce palliative care measures such as syringe drivers or morphine based analgesia early on could create conflict not only between physicians and carers but within those groups. Refusing to commence analgesia can be justified by the uncertainty of the prognosticated dying trajectory in Margaret's case as opposed to Jack's cancer diagnosis. Yet in both these cases, carers recognized pain and asked the physicians to increase the dosage. Familiarity with residents means that carers, with training, can learn how to recognize pain and deterioration not fully apparent in a quick clinical examination (Heath 2002). In neither case was an in-depth pain assessment undertaken at the first signs of deterioration. The response might be seen as reactive rather than pro-active. Pain was poorly managed in Margaret's case as demonstrated by the last minute scramble to get MST suppositories. Margaret's move into 'palliative care mode' was delayed by a stalling by the 'key decision maker', the general practitioner (Travis *et al.* 2001).

However, several aspects of good practice in end-of-life symptom control were evident. This included assessment of Jack's and Margaret's needs, physical contact from carers, including oral washes and turning as required as well as constant verbal reassurance that they were not alone.

The staff acknowledged that although they did not have nursing qualifications they felt comfortable giving 'nursing type care' as long as they were supported by the doctor and the district nurses. The case notes indicated the extent to which carers conveyed information about analgesia to one another—for example, side effects were noted as well as explanations for choices of drugs. Carers were willing to administer morphine and other types of analgesia. Their medication charts were easy to use. Yet in both these cases, carers felt frustrated by their 'failure' to address the resident's discomfort. Consequently the involvement of a palliative care link nurse or specialist palliative care team *as soon as the resident was seen to deteriorate* might have created a more seamless transition from conventional methods used in homes often referred to as 'tender loving care' to a more pro-active palliative care mode. This partnership could build confidence amongst home-based carers.

Communication

Keeping channels of communication open in relation to dying residents is a central tenet of palliative care, as well as being specified in most documents recommending care practices with all people, regardless of age or nearness to death. Communicating with (and about) residents should be a continual process, from admission throughout their stay in the home. Particularly when a resident is failing it is important to ensure that that person is informed and can participate, where possible, in decisions about care. Communication is therefore an on-going process even when it is unclear the extent to which a resident can understand verbal interactions.

(a) Between care staff and dying residents

Fundamental to the paradigm of palliative care is the belief that effective pain control is not possible without good communication. It is also essential to acknowledge the emotional needs of dying people. Dying people experience a variety of psychological changes, and symptoms may include some of those exhibited by Jack, fear, anxiety, and probably depression. Almost invariably dying people experience different forms of loss; these might include ability to feed oneself or communicate or other areas which are perceived as infringing their dignity, such as loss of continence. These emotions will impact on the relationship between dying person and the carer.

Good communication is based on upon sensitive listening and observation skills and an assessment of the resident's information needs. Care staff in Everglades were proud of the strong relationships that they developed with residents. They had an intuitive concept of the 'awareness contexts' (Glaser and Strauss 1965) exhibited by Jack who 'knew' he had cancer although he suspected the wrong kind. The carers believed that Jack was not keen to talk about his illness except to the doctor. They found this quite appropriate. However there was no evidence that carers gave Jack the openings he might have wanted to talk about his illness and impending death. Jack's sister Ann, reported that Jack demonstrated great distress particularly in relation to hoping to make peace with his ex-wife; carers reported that he seemed agitated following the visits of his children. However no action was taken to see whether talking about these issues might have created some relief for him.

Margaret's possible dementia and certain speech difficulties precluded discussions with her and in particular excluded her participation in any decision making. A central feature of palliative care is enabling dying people to exert choice and control. This is more difficult with the mentally frail. But Margaret's carers tried to include her in their conversations about her care—explaining what they were doing and providing comfort. Discussions about Margaret's care were carried out in her earshot, therefore if she were conscious she would have been aware that the carers thought she was dying.

Jack had made a decision to enter the home willingly after a trial period. Early in his dying trajectory he made choices about attempting to alleviate his shoulder pain by seeing a private physiotherapist and acquiring a TENS machine. The case notes suggest that Jack has consulted him about his preferred place of death (11.3). They also demonstrate that the GP chose to disclose information about his illness to Jack but in a measured way and based on his intimate knowledge of Jack. Jack was aware that the doctor discussed his situation with his children. A team approach which had included the key doctor(s), the carers, and the district nurse may have alleviated some of the uncertainty about who knew what and made Jack feel more in control of his dying.

(b) Amongst care staff and between care staff and outside professionals—multi-professional working

Everglades provides an example of good practice in relation to communication amongst care staff. Carers are notified formally and informally about a resident's condition—formal routes are institutionalized as part of what is perceived to be good professional practice. The emotional needs of carers were acknowledged in terms of requiring support to carry out demanding tasks as a resident approached death and died. Carers were also assumed to need support when someone died and this was provided in an informal way by phone or having a chat and weep in the kitchen. Expressing emotions was seen as natural and expected, but should not prevent carers from getting on with the job of caring for the living residents.

Carers, particularly management had strong opinions about the capabilities of the primary care teams that visited. Jack and Margaret belonged to different practices—in the one practice the doctors were not averse to setting up syringe drivers in care homes, in contrast to the other practice. However, Dr Reynolds stated that he probably would have responded to the home's request that he prescribe a syringe driver for Margaret once the suspension was not effective, rather than the suppositories prescribed by his partner, Dr Long. He felt that you can increase the dose and give a diamorphine boost quickly. He would have involved a district nurse to set it up and monitor it once a day as had been the case with Jack.

Neither GP practice had ever requested support for a dying resident in a care home from the Macmillan nurse team, nor the symptom care team from the local hospice. Nor had the home staff ever referred a resident to a Macmillan nurse but were not averse to this concept. Managers can 'educate' the primary care team in this respect, whilst acknowledging the sensitive nature of the relationship between community nurses who might feel deskilled by specialist palliative care nurses. The same applies to palliative care physicians and consultants in pain control who might have been able to make a positive contribution to both Jack and Margaret's care.

(c) Between care staff and residents' relatives

Supporting relatives and friends emotionally and enabling them to participate in the care of dying residents is central to palliative care. Many care homes already do this, although it is apparent that the roles of relatives depend on many factors—their relationship with and accessibility to the home, their prior relationships with the residents, the mental state of the resident and so forth. Some relatives want to fully participate in the physical care of the dying resident and this can have implications for staff's professional decision making (see Chapter 6). Communication training can help staff understand some of the issues in relation to relatives—these may include exploring problems of collusion—'Mum shouldn't know she has Alzheimers'.

Although staff members usually go to funerals many homes do not feel that it is appropriate for a funeral to leave from the home or for other residents to attend (see Chapter 6). Everglade's manager explained that it would be inappropriate for Margaret's funeral to leave from the home, would upset the other residents, and the home did not have the facilities to deal with either the flowers or the funeral party. Sometimes the environment creates constraints, particularly when the only reception room is the residents' lounge. However more flexibility in relation to both residents attending funerals and funerals or memorial services taking place in the home are acknowledged to be good bereavement care (CPA 1996).

Impact of a death on care staff, residents, and relatives—bereavement care

Palliative care encompasses bereavement care for friends and family. As noted earlier, other residents and staff often perceive themselves as almost family members of residents. When a resident is dying, other residents can be curious or concerned about them and may want to sit with them (CPA 1996).

Assessing the mood and capacity of residents in the spirit of person-centred care (DH 2001) may avoid creating a tense atmosphere, which in itself is difficult to manage. It is also important to recognize the collegiality of residents particularly those who communicate with one another, and that withholding information from them infantalises them and does not give them the choice and opportunities to express their feelings. Some knowledge about theories and patterns of grief could equip carers with some sense of how to gauge the feelings of surviving residents.

In considering these issues it should be noted that Everglades is typical of many homes in the United Kingdom where the majority of residents are white British. In other homes there are *residents* from minority ethnic groups but more frequently, *carers* from other religious or cultural backgrounds. As the immigrant population ages within the next 20 years one can assume that many people from minority ethnic groups will reside and die in care homes. Interactions between residents, home staff, and external professionals will have to accommodate mutual respect and understanding for feelings, rituals, practices, and possibly unfamiliar family relationships. The same will apply to communicating with resident's families, friends, and representatives of their religious or ethnic communities.

Conclusion

These two case studies demonstrate issues in relation to end-of-life practice in a residential home particularly around communication issues, communication about pain relief, within the home, with residents, relatives, and other professionals. Some of the National Minimum Standards for Dying and Death were met. Others such as Standard 11.7 which states that *'The registered person ensures that staff and service users who wish to offer comfort to a service user who is dying are enabled and supported to do so'* were not clearly demonstrated. Those standards demonstrated by the case studies include care staff making every effort to ensure the service user receives appropriate attention and pain relief (11.2) (even though they were unsuccessful), involving the service user's family and friends (11.4), enabling the service user to remain in their own rooms (11.6), presence of relatives and friends (11.10) and in Margaret's case time was allowed for family and friends to pay their respects to her after death (part of 11.11).

The quality of the dying for both Jack and Margaret may have been improved had specialist palliative care services been available (11.8). Standard Two of National Service Framework for Older People (DoH 2001), such as focusing on person-centred care resembles many parts of Standard 11 of the National Minimum Standards. Aspects of this do resonate in these cases, for example, maintaining the privacy and dignity of the service user (11.5) (see Chapter 2).

The nature of these two cases did not raise some of the ethical dilemmas in relation to end-of-life issues which are likely to arise more and more frequently reflecting the mood in the wider society. These concern decisions over whether or not to prolong life, and how to respond to advance directives, both of which were noted as important in *A Better Home Life* (CPA 1996). Additionally neither case study demonstrates some of the difficulties incurred when carers' cultural, religious or ethnic backgrounds differ markedly from that of the residents. Enabling carers to recognize and respect these differences will facilitate a person-centred approach to caring for dying residents and improve the potential for the dying resident to retain some control in a dignified way.

As the previous chapter suggested, the lack of training in the principles and practices of palliative care deprives carers of being able to deliver the standard of care to which they aspire and indeed which will be demanded of them to meet the National Minimum Standards. Carers require training as well as self-confidence in order to judge how best to care for a dying resident and their relatives.

The next chapter explores the care of dying residents in nursing homes in the United States.

References

Addington-Hall, J.M. and Higginson, I.J. (2001) Discussion, in J.M. Addington-Hall and I.J. Higginson (eds) *Palliative Care for Non-Cancer Patients*. Oxford University Press, Oxford.

Addington-Hall, J.M. and Higginson, I.J. (Eds) (2001) *Palliative Care for Non-Cancer Patients*. Oxford University Press, Oxford.

Avis, M., Jackson, J.G., Cox, K., and Miskella, C. (1999) Evaluation of a project providing community palliative care support to nursing homes. *Health and Social Care in the Community*, 7(1), 32–8.

Centre for Policy on Ageing (1996) *A Better Home Life*. Centre for Policy on Ageing, London.

Clare, J. and De Bellis, J. (1997) Palliative care in South Australian nursing homes. *Australian Journal of Advanced Nursing*, 14(4), 21–8.

Department of Health (2001) *National Service Framework for Older People*. Department of Health, London.

Doyle, D. and Jeffrey, D. (2000) *Palliative Care in the Home*. Oxford University Press, Oxford.

Glaser, B.G. and Strauss, A. (1965) *Awareness of Dying*. Aldine Publishing Company, Chicago.

Glaser, B.G. and Strauss, A. (1968) *Time for Dying*. Aldine Publishing Company, Chicago.

Heath, I. (2002) Long term care for older people. *British Medical Journal*, 324, 1534–5.

James, N. and Field, D. (1992) The routinization of hospice: Bureaucracy and charisma. *Social Science and Medicine*, 34(12), 1363–75.

Katz, J.T., Komaromy. C., and Sidell, M. (1999) Understanding palliative care in residential and nursing homes. *International Journal of Palliative Nursing*, 5(2), 58–64.

Katz, J.T., Komaromy. C., and Sidell, M. (2000a) Death in homes: Bereavement needs of residents, relatives and staff. *International Journal of Palliative Nursing*, 6(6), 274–9.

Katz, J.T., Komaromy. C., and Sidell, M. (2000*b*) *Investigating the Training Needs in Palliative Care*. Unpublished report for the Department of Health.

Komaromy, C., Sidell, M., and Katz, J.T. (2000) The quality of terminal care in residential and nursing homes. *International Journal of Palliative Nursing*, **6**(4), 192–204.

Lawton, J. (1998) Contemporary hospice care: The sequestration of the unbounded body and 'dirty dying'. *Sociology of Health and Illness*, **20**(2), 121–43.

Maddocks, I. and Parker, D. (2001) Palliative care in nursing homes, in J.M. Addington-Hall and I.J. Higginson (eds) *Palliative Care for Non-Cancer Patients*. Oxford University Press, Oxford, 148–57.

Peace, S., Kellaher, L., and Willcocks, D. (1997) *Re-evaluating Residential Care*. Open University Press, Buckingham.

Townsend, J., Frank, A.O., Fermont, D., Dyer, S., Karran, O., and Walgrave, A. (1990) Terminal Cancer Care and patients' preference for place of death: A prospective study. *British Medical Journal*, **301**, 415–7.

Travis, S.S., Loving, G., McClanahan, F.I., and Bernard, M. (2001) Hospitalization patterns and palliation in the last year of life among residents in long-term care. *The Gerontologist*, **41**(2), 153–60.

Zerzan, J., Stearnes, S., and Hanson, L. (2000) Access to palliative care and hospice in nursing homes. *JAMA*, **284**(19), 2489–94.

Appendix: The Everglades Procedure on death of a resident

At Everglades we like to give residents peace of mind that this is their home until death, and they do not have to worry at the first sign of a physical/mental problem that they will be moved elsewhere. Wherever possible we will care for them in every way possible, using the support of GPs, nursing services, and of course, the family.

When death is imminent this care will be in the resident's own room and as dignified as possible.

When death occurs

1. Contact the resident's GP.
2. Record time of death and names of staff present at the time.
3. If manager or deputies are not on duty, whoever is on call should be informed in order that family, if not present, can be contacted.
4. Resident should be placed lying flat, face up in bed, and as dignified as possible.
5. After GP and family have been contacted, and death has been certified, then the undertaker should be called to remove the body (the family will normally specify which one to use).

Sudden death

1, 2, and 3 as above.

Contact the police if resident has not been seen by a GP for two weeks. *Resident must NOT be moved until the police have given permission.*

Other residents will be informed, as necessary, of the death by the management in a dignified and sympathetic manner.

Proprietors: Mr and Mrs F. Jones

Chapter 10

Dying in long-term care facilities in the United States

Miriam S. Moss, Sidney Z. Moss, and Stephen R. Connor

This chapter is concerned with dying in long-term care facilities in the United States. First, it will briefly describe the nursing home as a primary focus of long-term care, then review some recent literature on end-of-life in nursing homes, followed by an examination of hospice care as it interfaces with nursing homes, and finally raise some concerns that have a bearing on planning future directions that end-of-life care may take in nursing homes.

Nursing homes in the United States

There are about 17 000 nursing homes in the United States and their average capacity is 107 beds. Over half (55 per cent) are part of a nursing home chain, where the median number of homes is 20 (Gabrel and Jones 2000). Few are part of a continuing care retirement community (6 per cent). Two-thirds (67 per cent) of the nursing homes are proprietary for profit, 26 per cent voluntary non-profit, and 7 per cent are facilities operated under federal, state, or local government auspices (Strahan 1997). The nursing home in the United States exists in an elaborate regulatory system. Standards have been set by state and federal governments, that mandate a periodic standardized assessment on each resident including data on cognitive functioning, physical health and functioning, communication problems, and many other items. In addition, periodic government inspections of the nursing home cover topics such as record keeping, staff training procedures, staff-resident ratios, and physical plant.

The two major streams of government funding for nursing home care in the United States are Medicare and Medicaid. *Medicare* is a health insurance programme for persons aged 65 and over as well as for eligible disabled persons. It is administered by the US Social Security Administration and provides medical assistance in the nursing home essentially restricted to post-hospital

skilled nursing and/or rehabilitation. *Medicaid* is a state administered programme for the medically indigent and is the primary reimbursement source
for care in nursing homes. Eligibility for Medicaid is based upon medical and
financial necessity and varies somewhat by states. Most states set a $2000 max-
imum for financial assets with an annual average income amount of $17 784
(maximum) (Kassner and Shirley 2000). Almost all (96 per cent) nursing
facilities are covered by Medicare and Medicaid (Gabrel and Jones 2000) and
the government pays 62 per cent of nursing home bills (US Health Care
Financing Administration 2000).

A nursing home may be certified by Medicare and/or Medicaid, or licensed by
the state. Officially it has at least three beds but the average capacity is over 100
beds. Each facility must provide on-site supervision by a licensed nurse 24 h
a day, 7 days a week and it must have a minimum staffing pattern of 2.7 h patient
care each day. The medical model is central in US nursing facilities; indeed the
Requirements of Participation in Medicare state that, 'the resident receives care
and services to attain or maintain the highest practicable physical, mental, and
psychosocial well-being' (Code of Federal Regulations 2000). Overall, the goals of
care are 'to maintain or improve physical and mental function, eliminate or
reduce pain and discomfort, provide social involvement and recreational activities in a safe environment, reduce unnecessary hospitalizations and emergency
room use, and provide a dignified death' (Maddox *et al.* 2001: 750).

Characteristics of the residents

Most (91 per cent) nursing home residents are aged 65 and over and at the time
of the 1997 National Nursing Home Survey the average age of residents at
admission was 83 years (Gabrel and Jones 2000). During the decade prior to
1997, the age of nursing home residents at entry increased as did their needs for
assistance with activities of daily living, while the length of nursing home stays
decreased. In 1997, the average length of stay was 276 days, and 85 per cent
received assistance in bathing and dressing (Gabrel and Jones 2000). This pattern may reflect increased use of home care because more people are remaining
longer in their own homes in the community and only moving into nursing
homes when they are more frail. The changes may also result from the increased
use of assisted living facilities that provide fewer services and attract the less frail
elderly, as well as the increased use of nursing home facilities for rehabilitation.

Nursing home care

The quality of care in nursing homes is not optimal, despite government over-
sight, surveys, and public concern. One recent estimate indicates that over one
quarter of the nursing homes 'had serious or potentially life threatening

problems in delivery of care', and that problems in quality of care tended to persist over time, with a need to strengthen enforcement of federal quality standards (US General Accounting Office 1999). Standards of staffing include the regulation that care aides should be trained and certified; they are routinely referred to as Certified Nursing Assistants (CNAs). Additionally each staff member must attend 12 hours of mandatory inservice training annually. In spite of these regulations, it has been suggested that poor care is largely reflective of inadequate standards for staffing (Harrington 2001). The result is often inadequate numbers of staff, paid low wages, few benefits, and associated patterns of high turnover. This factor must be seen in combination with some reluctance of accrediting agencies to enforce sanctions when poor care persists.

The well-being of residents may also suffer. There is consistent evidence that pain is under-treated for residents in long-term care facilities (Sengstaken and King 1993; Ferrell et al. 1995; Bernabei et al. 1998). A recent national study reported a pattern of persistent pain, such that 41 per cent of the residents in pain at a first assessment were in severe pain two to six months later (Teno et al. 2001). Further it is estimated that nearly half of the residents reported to be in pain were not receiving adequate pain control (Teno et al. 2001). One-third (35 per cent) of the 400 nursing homes in a recent national study agreed that they had pain control problems with demented residents (Moss et al. 2002). In addition to the prevalence of pain at the end of life, other problems may include food refusal and choking. Yet Volicer and Hurley (1998) describe how eating difficulties can be managed by the use of pharmacological, dietary, and nursing strategies without requiring tube feeding.

End of life in nursing homes

In the United States the quality of life at the end of life in nursing homes has historically received little attention—by clinicians, by researchers, or by policy and regulatory agencies. This in part is a reflection of ageism, the tendency to ignore the effects of deaths of older persons, and the emphasis on *living* in nursing homes. There is an entrenched boundary between living and dying in the nursing homes (Hockey 1990). The emphasis on living leaves little room for consideration of end-of-life issues. In the United States this may well be a reflection of the minimal overlap of theory and research in the fields of gerontology and of thanatology. The theme of disenfranchised grief is basically rooted in nursing homes' failure to recognize the impact of dying and death of residents on staff, family, and surviving residents.

Standards of care have been set for hundreds of aspects of the nursing home (physical environment, staffing, services available, etc.) by the federal agency that administers public funds for much of the care of institutionalized elderly

(Centres for Medicare and Medicaid, CMS) and by a private peer review accrediting commission (Joint Commission on the Accreditation of Healthcare Organizations, JCAHO). Little attention, however, has been paid by policy and regulatory agencies to the end of life. Yet, currently in the United States, 20 per cent of deaths occur in a nursing home (Brock and Foley 1998) and over a decade ago, it was estimated that a large proportion of persons aged 65 and over (43 per cent) will enter a nursing home before they die (Kemper and Murtaugh 1991). This group of older persons is likely to increase in size.

In the United States most elderly persons who move to a nursing home will die in an institution—either a nursing home or a hospital (Merrill and Mor 1993). It has been estimated that 25–44 per cent of residents are hospitalized annually (Castle and Mor 1996) and a recent study of residents with dementia at the end of life found that one-fourth die in the hospital (Moss *et al.* 2002). Very few nursing home residents have advance directives that are specific enough to address whether or not they wish to be hospitalized (Miller *et al.* 2001*a*). However, some research has examined patterns of mortality for nursing home residents. For example, in a study of the last 90 days in the life of older persons, age was associated with greater length of nursing home stay: age 75–84 was 22 days, and age 85 and over 42 days (Brock and Foley 1998).

The terminal decline of residents with cancer is often characterized by relatively high functioning until close to death followed by a short period of rapid decline. However, the top ten health conditions of nursing home residents in the United States (dementia, heart disease, hypertension, arthritis, cerebrovascular accident, depression, diabetes mellitus, anaemia, allergies, and chronic obstructive pulmonary disease) do not include cancer (Krauss and Altman 1998). Rather chronic conditions such as congestive heart failure are the norm, and these often have a cyclical pattern of decline and improvement in health and functioning (Lynn *et al.* 1998). Thus, it is often difficult to predict life expectancy for nursing home residents.

Currently there are some attempts to identify factors associated with death of nursing home residents. The expectation is that this information would help to alert staff to identify health care proxies, to clarify the residents' treatment wishes, and to reassess the care plan to be congruent with the residents' changing situation (Engle and Graney 1993; Breuer *et al.* 1998; Flacker and Kiely 1998). There is increasing use of advance directives in nursing homes, in part as a result of the 1991 Patient Self-Determination Act (Castle and Mor 1998). This Act requires Medicare providers to inform patients of their rights to execute advance directives. Most States have 'Directive to Physicians' (living wills) and 'Durable Power of Attorney for Health Care Decisions'. Both could be valuable in the future if the person becomes unable to make decisions for him or her self. Overall, 58 per cent of nursing home residents in a 1996 national survey have some form of advance directive (Degenholtz and Lave 1999). This primarily specifies no cardio-pulmonary resuscitation (CPR) which is particularly selected by older, female, white, more highly educated, longer term nursing home residents.

The research evidence in this area is contradictory, however. O'Brien and her colleagues undertook an in-depth study of preferences for life sustaining treatment by nursing home residents. Over 400 residents in 49 nursing homes were studied to ascertain their understanding of life-sustaining measures. Only one in eight reported that they had discussed their advanced directives with health care providers and less than a third had discussed them with family. Many decisionally capable nursing home residents had strong wishes for technological interventions: 89 per cent wanted CPR in case of cardiac arrest and 33 per cent wanted enteral tube feedings even if they were unable to eat because of permanent brain damage (O'Brien et al. 1995).

The impact of advance directives on care is not clear. In a study of terminal care for residents with dementia in 400 nursing homes, it was found that regardless of advance directives, for almost one-third of the most recent deaths there was some disagreement about end-of-life care between family and staff, resident and staff, or resident and family (Moss et al. 2002). In addition, advance directives in resident records transferred to a hospital have been found to be poorly documented and unrecognized in the hospital (Morrison et al. 1997).

The impact of residents' deaths

There is little formal recognition of the impact of a resident's death on family, staff, and surviving residents. End-of-life care is focused on the dying resident and on the need to maintain daily routines. Efforts are often made to minimize the impact of a resident's death. Most nursing homes do not have memorial services, funerals, and other rituals marking the death of a resident. In a recent study, over three quarters of the nursing homes reported that they had no funeral on site in the past year, and the majority held no memorial service (Moss et al. 2002).

Family

A prospective study examined pre-death predictors of strain on adult children whose parent died after living in a nursing home (Pruchno et al. 1995). The research found that being a daughter and being more upset about the parent living in nursing home were associated with greater emotional upset after the death. Further, perception of greater cognitive impairment of the parent was associated with greater sense of relief at the end of suffering, however cognitive status was not subsequently associated with amount of sadness, the degree of persistent thoughts, or the quality of memories of the parent. In responding to the dying and death of a parent with dementia, adult children often try to normalize the parent's behaviour, value the meaning of the parent's life, and maintain a continuing bond with the parent (Moss *et al.* 1996). Others have found that guilt was reduced after a nursing home resident's death (Aneshensel *et al.* 1995). There is some evidence that compared with the impact of having a parent die after living in the community, the impact of having a parent die in a nursing home results in lower grief, lower expression of grief, more acceptance of the death and less strong ties with the parent after death (Moss *et al.* 1997). This is not to suggest that the parent's death in a nursing home is not a meaningful and emotionally laden experience.

After the death, nursing home staff provide little or no support for bereaved family members. A telephone survey of 121 nursing homes in Michigan reported that although 55 per cent sent sympathy cards after the death, 98 per cent of the nursing homes did not visit, make telephone calls to, or provide written material on bereavement to family members (Murphy *et al.* 1997).

Staff

Nursing assistants provide 90 per cent of the hands-on care to dying residents (Ouslander 1994). Some research has suggested that one of the primary reasons that staff remains on the job is the meaningfulness of their relationships and attachments to residents (Monahan and McCarthy 1992). Family-like ties between staff and resident are often highly salient. Yet, themes of 'professional distance' and control of emotions are present in many facilities. Although administrative and supervisory staff recognize the importance of meaningful attachments between caregiving staff and residents (Savishinsky 1991; Gubrium 1997), this is not well supported by agency policy (Wilson and Daley 1998).

Staff often does not recognize some residents' concern about death, and avoid talking about the end of life with residents (Tellis-Nyack 1988). Staff's tendency towards covertness and silence around issues of dying and death may be seen as their way to protect residents and themselves from experiencing emotional upset. This may result in a disenfranchisement of staff emotional expression both before and after a resident's death (Moss and Moss 2002). Nursing home administrators have frequently recognized that facility support of bereaved staff needs improvement (Moss *et al.* 2002).

Major research efforts to explore the ways that direct-care staff perceive and behave in relation to end of life of nursing home residents is sparse. A major exception is the work in 28 nursing homes by Chichin and her colleagues (Chichin *et al.* 2000). They found that many nursing assistants (42 per cent) agree that if you talk to residents about a Do Not Resuscitate order, then they will think their condition is hopeless. Over half of the nursing assistants indicate that at times they have to act against their conscience in giving care to residents who are terminally ill. Many (42 per cent) say that staff who are caring for residents who are dying 'never' get emotional support or counselling. The medical model of staff training tends to emphasize the prolongation of life and the provision of life sustaining treatments, and the palliative model is of significantly less importance.

Surviving residents

Some residents prefer to have a dying roommate moved elsewhere and others prefer to keep close contact to see and comfort the dying resident (Lavigne-Pley and Levesque 1992). One nursing home was described as informing other residents when peers are failing in order to encourage them to say farewell (Bonifazi 1998). Often, however, the uncertainty of the timing of death deters prediction of death. After the death it is rare to have surviving residents spend time with the body. Generally, the facility conceals the body as it is removed and further has no formal way of communicating information on resident deaths. Nursing homes do not typically encourage families to have funeral services on site to allow residents and staff to attend.

Staff tends to pay little attention to the grief of surviving residents, perhaps in part because the staff's own grief is disenfranchised (Moss and Moss 2002). The grief of surviving residents tends to be disenfranchised not only by staff but also by family and residents themselves. When a deceased resident and a bereaved resident are both very old and frail, grief is doubly disenfranchised (Moss and Moss 1989).

Interface between hospice and nursing homes

Historically, hospice developed in the United States as an alternative to aggressive medical treatment in a hospital environment. Hospice focused on providing palliative care by an interdisciplinary team. The goal was to provide enough support, both physical and psychosocial, that the patients would be able to remain in their homes while going through the dying process, surrounded by their family and friends. Cancer patients were the initial focus of hospice care and today in the United States they still represent the largest category of hospice recipients. In 2000, 57 per cent of hospice admissions were for cancers while the remaining 43 per cent included patients with heart and lung diseases, dementias, kidney and liver disease, HIV, stroke/coma, and motor neuron disease (National Hospice and Palliative Care Organization 2002).

There has been increasing emphasis in the hospice movement to move beyond a primary focus on care for terminally ill cancer patients to persons with non-cancer diseases. In recent years the National Hospice Organization (now named the National Hospice and Palliative Care Organization) has begun to delineate guidelines to facilitate referrals to hospice of persons with non-cancer diseases such as chronic pulmonary disease and Alzheimer's Disease (National Hospice Organization 1996).

After a series of research studies that focused on the feasibility of including hospice as an option for federal reimbursement, the Medicare hospice benefit was established in 1982 both to improve the quality of care for the dying and as a mechanism for potential cost saving. The Omnibus Budget Reconciliation Act of 1989 clarified that 'there is no indication in the statute that the term 'home' is to be limited for a hospice patient. A patient's home is where he or she resides. The facility is considered to be the beneficiary's place of residence (the same as a house or apartment), and the facility resident may elect the hospice benefit if he/she also meets the hospice eligibility criteria' (State Operations Manual, Section 2082, 1998). This allowed Medicare to reimburse hospice services to nursing home residents.

Throughout the subsequent development of the interface between hospice and nursing homes, regulatory processes for nursing homes have been, and continue to be, more developed, detailed and in place than regulations for hospices. The partnership between hospice and nursing facility providers is only addressed in the 'Surveyor Guidelines' in the State Operations Manual. Although guidelines for both are similar in many ways, there are differences, that create confusion and a lack of clarity. Both providers are held to their own Conditions of Participation from a regulatory perspective.

The interface between nursing homes and hospices is an increasing phenomenon in the United States. Although only 1 per cent of nursing homes have a hospice unit sponsored by the nursing home (Petrisek and Mor 1999), almost three quarters (72 per cent) of nursing homes report that, through outside providers, they offer to bring in services provided by hospice organizations in the community (Gabrel and Jones 2000).

To receive hospice benefits under Medicare, nursing home residents must be eligible for Medicare and be certified by their physician to have a life expectancy of six months or less if their disease runs its normal course. Hospice provides a range of services from an interdisciplinary team composed of physician, nurse, aide, social worker, clergy, volunteers, and therapists. In addition, out-patient medications, medical supplies, and medical equipment that are related to the terminal illness are also covered without payment from the Medicare recipient. At the same time, patients receiving hospice waive their right to receive standard Medicare benefits for treatment of their terminal condition including curative treatments, such as hospitalization, home health benefit, and skilled nursing home benefit.

In general, the hospice is reimbursed a per diem rate under the prospective reimbursement system at the same rate as for patients in their homes. For Medicaid recipients in nursing homes, the hospice receives an additional amount equal to 95 per cent of the rate that would have been paid the facility. Under a contractual arrangement, the hospice then pays the nursing facility for room and board which includes the following:

- performing personal care services
- assisting with activities of daily living
- administering medication
- socializing activities
- maintaining cleanliness of a resident's room
- supervising and assisting in the use of durable medical equipment and prescribed therapies.

A major investigation was undertaken by the federal government to examine the extent to which hospice patients living in nursing homes may have been admitted to hospice with inappropriate diagnosis and were living extended periods of time (US Office of the Inspector General 1997). Results of this investigation did not find fraud or waste to be a significant concern, however the Office of the Inspector General continues to be concerned about payment for hospice care in nursing facilities. A study commissioned by the US Department of Health and Human Services has subsequently found that hospitalization rates in the last 30 days of life are lower when hospice care is provided in a nursing facility. The greater the hospice presence in a nursing home, the lower the hospital use for all dying residents in the nursing home (Miller et al. 2001a). Further, in a study of nursing home residents with daily pain, it was found that hospice recipients were twice as likely to receive regular treatment for daily pain, than matched non-hospice controls (Miller et al. 2002).

Another landmark study to estimate the use of hospice in nursing homes utilized multiple data sources routinely provided by almost 17 000 nursing homes and by over 2000 hospices (Petrisek and Mor 1999). Overall Petrisek and Mor (1999) found that nursing homes with the larger concentration of patients receiving hospice benefits were more likely to be for-profit, to have greater nurse staffing ratios, and a higher percentage of residents receiving pain management. Further, Petrisek and Mor examined market and environmental characteristics associated with hospice use in nursing homes. Greater hospice use was reported in nursing homes located in urban counties, with more competitive nursing home markets, and more for-profit hospices. States and regions in the United States differed considerably in providing hospice care to nursing home residents. Overall, Petrisek and Mor suggest that 'the distribution of Medicare hospice beneficiaries in nursing homes does follow an economically motivated path because the factors associated with this organizational behaviour could be interpreted as an attempt to maximize reimbursement' (p. 289). They emphasize that the hospice benefit potentially plays a crucial role in ensuring effective pain control and compliance with resident's wishes at the end of life.

There is little or no financial incentive for the nursing home to include hospice care. The attitudes of nursing home administrators can play a major role in the extent that a facility uses hospice (Jones *et al.* 1997). Direct care staff provided by hospice can reduce the potential burdens on the nursing home staff to provide needed one-on-one care at the end of life. The value of the palliative care skills provided by hospice are particularly relevant in the domain of pain and symptom control.

Some community residents who have received hospice subsequently move to a nursing home where they continue to receive hospice care. Recently it has been estimated that they represent about 10 per cent of all nursing home hospice recipients (Miller and Mor 2001). No research has examined how this process takes place, and how the staff of hospice and nursing homes facilitate this transition.

Further we do not know who initiates the idea of hospice care for terminally ill residents. It may be that the physician or nurse initiates the discussion of hospice. As hospice care becomes more prominent in communities, patient/family members may initiate the referral process based on previous experiences with others. As hospice becomes more recognized as a treatment option at the end of life for non-cancer patients, family and resident requests may be expected to increase.

Once hospice care begins it does not always continue until death. Of nursing homes with hospice available in a recent national survey, 18 per cent indicated that within the past 12 months one or more residents with advanced dementia had been discharged from hospice back to regular nursing care (Moss *et al.* 2002). This tends to reflect stabilization or even improvement in the resident's condition, often attributed to the hospice care received.

Extent of hospice use in nursing homes

The proportion of Medicare hospice beneficiaries living in a nursing home has been increasing from 8 per cent of all in 1989, to 17 per cent in 1995 (Zerzan *et al.* 2000), to the most recent estimate of 24 per cent in 1996 (Miller and Mor 2001). The prospect of a nursing home resident receiving hospice care, however, is very low. Petrisek and Mor found that on the day of their survey only 1 per cent of residents received hospice care; 70 per cent of the nursing homes reported that they had no residents receiving Medicare hospice benefits on that day. In one major study of nursing homes, it was reported that only 1.3 per cent of nursing home residents aged 65 and over had received hospice service during the 30 days prior to the survey (Gabrel and Jones 2000). Overall, it has been estimated that five or six percent of all dying nursing home residents have received hospice care (Keay and Schonwetter 1998; Miller and Mor 2001). The average length of hospice care for nursing home residents was 90.6 days, the median 35 days, and the mode two days (Miller and Mor 2001).

It is difficult to evaluate the impact of hospice use in facilities such as nursing homes. It is challenging to disentangle the influence of hospice care *vis-à-vis* the characteristics of the nursing home that chooses hospice. Further, even within a facility comparing hospice cases with non-hospice cases, research must consider the likely impact of a 'spill over' effect which may mask the impact of hospice (Miller *et al.* 2001b). There is some evidence that staff feels that the presence of hospice positively influences the care of non-hospice dying residents. The above mentioned research comparing nursing home deaths with and without hospice in terms of the appropriateness of pain medication, and the likelihood of hospitalization have attempted to deal with this confound.

Barriers to hospice use in nursing homes

Barriers to hospice in nursing homes are numerous. A significant factor is the difficulty of determining a terminal, six month prognosis. It is particularly difficult to identify a risk profile to reliably estimate the life expectancy of patients with dementia (Luchins *et al.* 1997; Volicer and Hurley 1998; Gambassi *et al.* 1999). There is some evidence that the severity of dementia itself has no influence on survival (Gambassi *et al.* 1999).

Perhaps one of the major barriers is that the nursing home staff, both administrative and caregiving, have been committed to the ongoing care of each resident. Nursing home staff usually knows the resident over a period of months or years and often has developed a strong bond. Staff takes pride in knowing resident preferences, in being able to recognize subtle changes and signs of discomfort, and in knowing the resident's family members. Staff has an expectation that they can provide continuity in caregiving, and meet the resident's needs. They may subtly see the potential entry of another service team as an indication that their power and competence is diminished.

Another potential barrier may be from physicians who resist having other caregivers with whom they must collaborate in resident care. Further, some nursing homes may resist hospice for fiscal reasons: for example, if reimbursement through hospice is not equal to the normal third-party payments the nursing home would receive for more skilled nursing care. A resident who is receiving the Medicare skilled nursing benefit cannot receive the Medicare hospice benefit at the same time. In addition, nursing home administrators may fear that inspectors will negatively evaluate weight loss, reduced functioning, and other characteristics of dying residents, failing to account for a normal terminal trajectory. Finally, a barrier may be rooted in the resistance of family members who are unwilling to face the end of life of their relative.

In light of the above barriers, it is not surprising that when one study asked 'In order to be eligible for hospice services, the life expectancy of the resident must be six months or less. *Not* counting those currently receiving hospice, how many current residents are now eligible for hospice?' In two thirds of the nursing homes where hospice was available, four or more additional residents were judged as eligible for hospice (Moss *et al.* 2002).

Best practices of nursing homes and hospices

Another study also examined attitudes of nursing homes towards hospice care and attitudes of hospice towards their care for nursing home residents (Moss *et al.* 1999). Specifically it focused on end-of-life care for elders with dementia. Nationally the proportion of nursing home residents with dementia has been estimated to be between half and three-quarters. We know, however, of no recent research that estimates the prevalence of dementia at the end of life for nursing home residents.

Ninety nursing homes that participated in the above national survey were matched with 90 hospices that provided care to residents of these nursing homes. Thus, the paired agencies are from the same communities, serving similar client groups. This study found that most nursing homes (87 per cent) do not formally orient hospice staff in how to care for residents with dementia, while most hospices (71 per cent) do provide their staff with in-service training on this topic. Although hospices report that they give 'excellent' care for the dying nursing home residents who are cognitively alert (92 per cent), fewer report that they give this level of care to dying residents with advanced dementia (64 per cent).

The above study asked hospices and nursing homes to indicate three things that they do best. Strong similarities as well as differences emerged. There were no differences in such best practices as keeping the resident comfortable, emotional support for the dying resident, keeping close contact with the family.

About half (49 per cent) of nursing homes selected as a best practice 'staff treats resident like family', while this was judged a best practice by only 6 per cent of the hospices. Additionally, nursing homes more frequently indicated best practices included continuity of caregivers. When reporting on the practices they do 'least well' hospices more often than nursing homes, reported emotional support for other residents. Nursing homes more often than hospices reported spiritual care, staff training around death and around pain control as 'least well' performed.

The above differences may suggest that the ideology of the nursing home is not very strongly influenced by the hospice, and vice versa. It further may reflect their basic differences in orientation to resident care, and suggest potential problems in their working relationships.

Perspectives on the future

Overall the cultural and policy milieu in the United States seems to be changing slowly towards some increased acceptance of palliative care at the end of life in nursing homes. There is a tradition for nursing homes in the United States to provide care for older persons towards the end of their lives, most often up to the moment of death. Although hospice is available through many nursing homes, it is not clear that these long-term care facilities have embraced the potential of integrating hospice care into their milieu. In the future, barriers to hospice care may decrease as the pain and symptom control skills of hospice and the broader palliative care model become more integrated into long-term care.

The question repeatedly arises: what is the difference between normal nursing home care and nursing home care at the end of life? Both are concerned with maximizing psychological well-being and functional status, meeting religious and spiritual needs, pain and symptom control, communication of advance directives, giving residents maximal control over the way they live and the way they die. Careful consideration of this issue may be productive.

There are strengths and weaknesses of regulatory approaches to quality as well as of market approaches to quality. As alluded to above, there is some concern by nursing homes about the ways that regulatory and accreditation bodies evaluate end-of-life care. Currently issues of comfort do not take precedence over traditional concerns around pressure ulcers, hydration, and weight loss. There is little incentive for nursing homes to integrate the palliative care model when they find themselves caught between their need to meet regulatory standards and their need to provide appropriate end-of-life care.

In the United States, the medical model of care tends to be paramount in long-term care. When emotional, social, and spiritual aspects of quality of life are added to the physical needs of the resident, it may be possible to evaluate the overuse of interventions as well as the under use of effective services (Donaldson 1998).

Finally we must continue to view end-of-life care in nursing homes within the changing context of demography and policy. As nursing homes take on more rehabilitation and subacute care functions, and concomitantly while home care and assisted living facilities are increasingly available to the elderly, there will potentially be more elderly who are more frail with shorter stays in nursing homes. In the future, the nursing home may well continue to be the place of death for many elderly persons. Issues of quality of care and quality of life at the end of life will become increasingly central.

Research findings and policy developments concerning end-of-life issues in long term care are being seen in both the United Kingdom and the United States. It is hoped that each country can benefit from a careful consideration of the policy, practices, and research of the other.

References

Aneshensel, C.S., Pearlin, L.I., Mullan, J.T., Zarit, S.H., and Whitlatch, C.J. (1995) *Profiles in Caregiving: The Unexpected Career* Academic Press, San Diego, CA.

Bernabei, R., Gambassi, G., Lapane, K. *et al.* (1998) Management of pain in elderly patients with cancer. *Journal of the American Medical Association*, 279, 1877–82.

Bonifazi, W. (1998) Final acts. *Contemporary Long Term Care*, 21, 52–61.

Breuer, B., Wallenstein, S., Feinberg, C., Camargo, M.-J.F., and Libow, L.S. (1998) Assessing life expectances of older nursing home residents. *Journal of the American Geriatrics Society*, 46, 954–62.

Brock, D.B. and Foley, D.J. (1998) Demography and epidemiology of dying in the US with emphasis on deaths of older persons. *Hospice Journal*, 13, 49–60.

Castle, N.G. and Mor, V. (1996) Hospitalization of nursing home residents: A review of the literature, 1980–1995. *Medical Care Research and Review*, 53, 123–48.

Castle, N.G. and Mor, V. (1998) Advance care planning in nursing homes: Pre- and post-patient self-determination act. *Health Services Research*, 33, 101–24.

Chichin, E.R., Burack, O.R., Olson, E., and Likourezos, A. (2000) *End-of Life Ethics and the Nursing Assistant*. Springer, New York.

Code of Federal Regulations (2000) *Quality of Care*, vol. 42, 483.25.

Degenholtz, H.B. and Lave, J. (1999) *Predictors of Advance Directives Among Nursing Home Residents*. Paper presented at the Annual Meeting in November 1999 of the Gerontological Society of America, San Francisco.

Donaldson, M.S. (1998) The importance of measuring quality of care at the end of life. *Hospice Journal*, 13, 1117–38.

Engle, V.F. and Graney, M.J. (1993) Predicting outcomes of nursing home residents: Death and discharge home. *Journal of Gerontology: Social Sciences*, 48, 269–75.

Ferrell, B.A., Ferrell, B.R., and Rivera, L. (1995) Pain in cognitive impaired nursing home patients. *Journal of Pain Symptom Management*, 10, 591–8.

Flacker, J.M. and Kiely, D.K. (1998) A practical approach to identifying mortality-related factors in established long term care residents. *Journal of the American Geriatric Society*, 46, 1012–15.

Gabrel, C. and Jones, A. (2000). The national nursing home survey: 1997 Summary. US National Center for Health Statistics. *Vital Statistics*, 13, 147.

Gambassi, G., Landi, F., Lapane, K.L., Sgadari, A., Mor, V., and Bernabei, R. (1999) Predictors of mortality in patients with Alzheimer's disease living in nursing homes. *Journal of Neurological Neurosurgical Psychiatry*, 67, 59–65.

Gubrium, J.F. (1997) *Living and Dying at Murray Manor*. University Press of Virginia, Charlottesville, VA.

Harrington, C. (2001) Residential nursing facilities in the United States. *British Medical Journal*, 323, 507–10.

Hockey, J.L. (1990) *Experiences of Death: An Anthropological Account*. Edinburgh University Press, Edinburgh, Scotland.

Jones, B., Nackerud, L., and Boyle, D. (1997) Differential utilization of hospice services in nursing homes. *Hospice Journal*, 12, 41–57.

Kassner, E. and Shirley, L. (2000) *Medicaid Financial Eligibility for Older People: State Variations in Access to Home and Community-Based Waiver and Nursing Home Services*. Public Policy Institute, AARP, Washington, DC.

Keay, T.J. and Schonwetter, R.S. (1998) Hospice care in the nursing home. *American Family Physician*, 57, 491–4.

Kemper, P. and Murtaugh, C.M. (1991) Lifetime use of nursing home care. *New England Journal of Medicine*, 324, 595–600.

Krauss, N.A. and Altman, B.M. (1998) *Characteristics of nursing home residents—1996*. Rockville, MD: Agency for Health Care Policy and Research. MEPS Research Findings No. 5. AGCPR Pub. No. 99-0006.

Lavigne-Pley, C. and Levesque, L. (1992) Reactions of the institutional elderly upon learning of the death of a peer. *Death Studies* 16, 451–61.

Luchins, D.J., Hanrahan, P., and Murphy, K. (1997) Criteria for enrolling dementia patients in hospice. *Journal of the American Geriatrics Society*, 45, 1054–9.

Lynn, J., Wilkinson, A., Cohn, F., and Jones, S.B. (1998) Capitated risk-bearing managed care systems could improve end-of-life care. *Journal of the American Geriatrics Society*, 46, 322–30.

Maddox, G.L. *et al.* (2001). *The Encyclopedia of Aging*. (3rd edition) Springer, New York.

Merrill, D. and Mor, V. (1993) Pathways to hospital death among the oldest old. *Journal of Aging and Health*, 5, 516–35.

Miller, S.C. and Mor, V. (2001) The emergence of Medicare hospice care in U.S. nursing homes. *Palliative Care*, 15, 471–80.

Miller, S.C., Gozalo, P., and Mor, V. (2001a) Hospice enrollment and hospitalization of dying nursing home patients. *American Journal of Medicine*, 111, 38–44.

Miller, S.C., Mor, V., Gage, B., and Coppola, K. (2001b) Hospice and its role in improving end-of-life care, in M.P. Lawton (ed.) *Focus on the End of Life: Scientific and Social Issues. Annual Review of Gerontology and Geriatrics*, 20, 193–223.

Miller, S., Mor, V., Wu, N., Gozalo, P., and Lapane, K. (2002) Does receipt of hospice care in nursing homes improve the management of pain at the end of life? *Journal of American Geriatrics Society*, 50, 507–15.

Monahan, R. and McCarthy, S. (1992) Nursing home employment: The nurses aide perspective. *Journal of Gerontological Nursing*, 18, 13–116.

Morrison, R.S., Olson, E., Mertz, K.R., and Meier, D.E. (1997) The inaccessibility of advance directives on transfer from ambulatory to acute care settings. *Journal of the American Medical Association*, 274, 478–82.

Moss, M.S., Braunschweig, H., and Rubinstein, R.L. (1999). *Hospice Care for Nursing Home Residents with Dementia: Hospice and Nursing Home Perspectives*. Poster presented at Annual Meeting Gerontological Society of America, Philadelphia, PA.

Moss, M.S., Braunschweig, H., and Rubinstein, R.L. (2002) Terminal care for nursing home residents with dementia. *Alzheimer Care Quarterly*, 3, 233–46.

Moss, M.S. and Moss, S.Z. (1989) Death of the very old, in K. Doka (ed.) *Disenfranchised Grief: Recognizing Hidden Sorrow*. Lexington Books, Lexington, MA, 213–27.

Moss, S.Z. and Moss, M.S. (2002) Nursing home staff reactions to resident Deaths, in K. Doka (ed.) *Disenfranchised Grief: New Directions*. Research Press, Champaign, IL, 197–216.

Moss, S.Z., Moss, M.S., and Rubinstein, R.L. (1996) *Death of a parent Who Lived in a Nursing Home*. Paper presented at the Annual Meeting in November 1996 of the Gerontological Society of America, Washington, DC.

Moss, M.S., Resch, N., and Moss, S.Z. (1997) The role of gender in middle aged children's responses to parent death. *Omega*, 35, 43–65.

Murphy, K., Hanrahan, P., and Luchins, D. (1997) A survey of grief and bereavement in nursing homes. *Journal of American Geriatric Society*, 45, 1104–7.

National Hospice and Palliative Care Organization (2002). Facts and figures on hospice care in America. Retrieved 5-2-2002 from www.nhpco.org National Hospice Organization (1996) *Medical Guidelines for Determining Prognosis in Selected Non-Cancer Diseases*. (2nd edition) Arlington, VA.

O'Brien, L.A., Grisso, J.A., Maislin, G., LaPann, K., Krotki, K.P., Greco, P.J., Siegert, E.A., and Evans, L.K. (1995) Nursing home residents' preferences for life-sustaining treatments. *Journal of the American Medical Associaton*, 274, 1775–9.

Ouslander, J.G. (1994) Nursing home care, in W. Hazzard (ed.), *Principles of Geriatric Medicine and Gerontology*. (3rd edition) McGraw Hill, New York.

Petrisek, A.C. and Mor, V. (1999) Hospice in nursing homes: A facility-level analysis of the distribution of hospice beneficiaries. *The Gerontologist*, 39, 279–90.

Pruchno, R.A., Moss, M.S., Burant, C.J., and Schinfeld, S. (1995) Death of an institutionalized parent: Predictors of bereavement. *Omega*, 31, 99–119.

Savishinsky, J.S. (1991) *The Ends of Time*. Bergin and Garvey, New York.

Sengstaken, E.A. and King, S.A. (1993) The problems of pain and its detection among geriatric nursing home residents. *Journal of the American Geriatrics Society*, 41, 541–4.

Strahan, G.W. (1997) *An Overview of Nursing Homes and their Current Residents: Data from the 1995 National Nursing Home Survey*. (Advance Data from Vital and Health Statistics, No. 280.) National Center for Health Statistics, Hyattsville, MD.

State Operations Manual, Section 2082 (1998) *Election of hospice benefit by resident of SNF, NF, ICF/MR or non-certified facility*.

Tellis-Nayak, V. (1988) *Nursing Home Exemplars of Quality*. C.C. Thomas, Springfield, IL.

Teno, I.M., Weitzen, S., Wetle, T., and Mor, V. (2001) Persistent pain in nursing home residents. *Journal of American Medical Association*, 285, 2081.

US General Accounting Office (1999) *Nursing homes: Additional steps needed to strengthen enforcement of federal quality standards*. GAO, Washington DC. (Report to the Special Committee on Aging, US Senate.)

US Health Care Financing Administration (2000) *National Health Expenditures (1960–98)*. HCFA, Washington, DC.

US Office of the Inspector General (1997) *Hospice Patients in Nursing Homes*. (DHHS Publication No. OE1-05-95-002450). Department of Health and Human Services, Washington, DC.

Volicer, L. (1998) Tube feeding in Alzheimer's disease is avoidable. *Research in Alzheimer's Disease*, 1, 71–4.

Volicer, L. and Hurley, A. (1998) *Hospice Care for Patients with Advanced Progressive Dementia*. Springer, New York.

Wilson, S.A. and Daley, B.I. (1998) Attachment/detachment: Forces influencing care of the dying in long term care. *Journal of Palliative Medicine*, 1, 21–34.

Zerzan, I., Stearns, S., and Hanson, L. (2000) Access to palliative care and hospice in nursing homes. *Journal of American Medical Association*, 284, 2489–94.

Chapter 11

Issues for palliative care in nursing and residential homes

David Field and Katherine Froggatt

Introduction

In the United Kingdom, as elsewhere (Maddocks and Parker 2001), nursing and residential homes have become increasingly important locations for the care of people who are dying. In 1993 Field and James estimated that the 12–15 per cent of people dying in the United Kingdom did so in nursing and residential homes. Since that time these sectors have continued to expand and current estimates are that this proportion has risen to just under 19 per cent in England and Wales. In this chapter we will identify and discuss the main issues concerned with providing palliative care to older people living in nursing and residential care homes in the United Kingdom. Before doing so we briefly review the social and policy context that has made the care of people dying in such Homes an important issue. More detailed discussion will be found in Chapters 1 and 2. Where appropriate, we will differentiate between nursing and residential homes in our discussion. It should be noted that there is relatively little research about the care of dying people in UK care homes and that most of this refers to nursing homes.

Defining palliative care in nursing and residential homes

There is some understandable confusion about what is meant by the term 'palliative care'. The most widely quoted definition is provided by the World Health Organisation (1990): 'the active total care of patients and families by a multi-professional team when the patient's disease is no longer responsive to curative treatment'. However, in practice the ideal of delivering palliative care by a multi-professional *team* is still the exception rather than the rule, even when a number of health care professionals are involved in delivering care to those who are dying. The National Council for Hospice and Specialist Palliative Care Services (NCHSPCS 1995) distinguishes between specialist palliative care services and a more general 'palliative care approach', aiming 'to promote both physical and psychosocial well being'. Palliative care will encompass both of these and be provided by both generalists (e.g. general practitioners and community nurses), and specialists in palliative care (e.g. Macmillan nurses, consultants in palliative medicine).

We saw in Chapter 1 that palliative care has developed from the care of cancer patients by hospice organizations and still caters mainly for cancer patients (Eve and Smith 1996). However, since the 1990s attention has increasingly turned to the provision of palliative care for people dying from non-malignant conditions, with the recognition that people with such conditions had unmet needs for palliative care (Field and Addington-Hall 1999). This has come to be known as 'generic palliative care', and refers to the adoption of a palliative care approach by other hospital based specialists and 'generalist' health professionals (district nurses, general practitioners, care home staff, etc.) working in the community.

Health and social policy

The current policy agendas in the arenas of cancer, cardiac, and older people's services will shape the delivery of palliative care to these care homes and reflect the diversification from specialist to generic palliative care in various ways. The Cancer Plan (DoH 2000*a*) addresses palliative care primarily through a Government commitment to increased funding for hospices and specialist palliative care services and investment in training and support for district nurses and other community based nurses. The latter initiative indicates an increasing emphasis on the delivery of palliative care in non-acute settings (domestic homes in the community) by general rather than specialist practitioners.

Another way in which the provision of palliative care is being broadened can be seen in the National Service Framework for Coronary Heart Disease (DoH 2000*b*). A consideration of the benefit palliative care services can bring to people with coronary heart disease is highlighted along with explicit mention of palliative care teams being a source of local support as needed. These recommendations are further emphasizing a model of care on the basis of need not diagnosis. This obviously has implications for the types of service provision required, as people with conditions other than cancer may not have the prognostic certainties usually present with the malignant disease progression and around which services have developed. As seen in Chapter 2 this particular model is also present in the National Service Framework for Older People (DoH 2001*b*), which promotes the provision of care and services that are responsive to individual need, regardless of where individuals are residing, be it at home, in residential care, or in hospital. The NSF explicitly recognizes that older people who live with chronic conditions or who are approaching the end of life may need supportive and palliative care (see Chapter 2: p. 39).

As outlined in the National Minimum Standards for Care Homes (DoH 2001a, Chapter 2: p. 37) the use of trained professionals or specialist agencies in palliative care for residents in care homes should occur if the service user so wishes.

Within these policy initiatives the provision of palliative and supportive care to older people and people living with non-malignant chronic conditions is encouraged. However, in reality how such care can be offered and delivered when required is problematic. A number of barriers to the extension of specialist palliative care to all those requiring it have been identified (Field and Addington-Hall 1999). For individuals to receive appropriate care when they need or desire it will require the issues concerning the boundaries of specialist and generic palliative care to be addressed with respect to patients, staff and service delivery. This is discussed in more detail below.

Both nursing and residential care homes provide care for older people, but they offer different types of care that meet the needs of different levels of dependency. As outlined in Chapter 2, residential homes have no requirement to employ registered nurses and carers, who may or may not have NVQ qualifications in social care, provide care although as already noted the National Minimum Standards for Care Homes have recommended that 50 per cent of care assistants should have achieved NVQ Level II by 2005 (DoH 2001a). Chapter 7 shows that the presence of registered nurses in nursing homes, but not residential care homes, affects the degree to which community nursing services are involved with residents dying in care homes: district nurses can be involved in the care of residents in residential care homes, but not nursing homes. General practitioners play a key role in the care of residents in both types of home (see Chapter 9). Nursing Homes can be registered to care for terminally ill people and/or designate registered palliative care beds provided they meet particular standards (NAHAT 1991). Designated beds in nursing homes can also be registered with the local health authority to provide palliative care for individuals assessed as requiring more specialist palliative care input.

The operationalization of the recommendations concerning the provision of palliative care regardless of diagnosis or care setting has yet to be addressed. In the case of the provision of palliative care in care homes a number of other issues also need to be recognized and will now be discussed.

Factors affecting the provision of palliative care in nursing and residential care homes

Two main features influence the way in which the provision of palliative care within nursing and residential care homes can be delivered: the people who are potential recipients of palliative care and the cultural and structural factors that shape how care is delivered within these settings. In practice, as our discussion reflects, these interact with each other.

The care home population

As discussed in Chapter 2, the care home population is a complex one because it is both homogeneous with respect to some demographic characteristics but heterogeneous with respect to the type of care required. It is the level of dependency, rather than biological age that determines the care status of particular residents. Older people who, for whatever reason, become unable to be self-supporting are viewed by society as a homogeneous group and sequestered away (Hockey 1990; Mellor and Shilling 1993; Froggatt 2001b). Care homes provide spaces to contain this separation (Hockey 1990; Peace et al. 1997). People *live* as well as die in care homes, so there is a particular tension when it comes to looking at palliative care or end-of-life care in these particular settings (as discussed in Chapter 2). As noted by a number of authors (Clark and Seymour 1999; Field 2000), within gerontological writing there is little evidence of attention to death and dying. Gerontological practice is primarily focused upon the care of the living and attaining their maximum capability whatever the age. The challenge is to provide, within the same institution, end-of-life care as well as good supportive care for both the 'fit' and the 'frail'.

Perhaps the most fundamental challenges to developing palliative care for residents is the pattern of morbidity and the nature of dying found in care homes. Residents in such homes as compared to those living in their own homes or those of relatives are more likely to:

- be suffering from chronic and long-term conditions
- have significantly greater restrictions of their activities
- have higher levels of mental confusion, incontinence, impaired sight, and hearing.

(Cartwright 1991; George and Sykes 1997; Maddocks and Parker 2001: 149–50)

Since the 1993 review by Field and James a small number of studies in the United Kingdom (Shemmings 1996; Sidell et al. 1997; Miskella and Avis 1998; Avis et al. 1999; Katz et al. 1999; Froggatt 2000; Lloyd 2000) have provided greater insight into the care of dying people in these settings. Of particular relevance for our discussion is the identification of the patterns of dying typically found in care homes. OU Study (1) (Sidell et al. 1997) found that 42 per cent of the deaths of residents in their large-scale study were the result of 'general deterioration'; in nursing homes over half of all deaths (51 per cent) fell into this category (see Chapter 3). Thirty-four per cent of deaths resulted from an acute episode, 6 per cent from sudden death and only 9 per cent from an already recognized terminal illness. The latter two types were more common in residential homes than in nursing homes (12 and 19 per cent, respectively). A small scale qualitative study of nursing homes by Froggatt (2001b) confirmed the high presence of deaths that were the result of a gradual general deterioration described by staff as 'going downhill' and as 'fading', 'failing', and 'lingering'. There was also a great deal of uncertainty present about whether or not people were actually dying (Froggatt 2001b). This pattern of dying contrasts to that found amongst people dying with malignancies and a few neurological conditions under the auspices of palliative care in a range of settings (hospitals, hospices, and domestic homes) and has important implications for identifying residents as dying and, hence, as eligible for or in need of palliative care (see Chapters 4 and 6).

A further key issue is that the majority of dying residents do so from chronic conditions other than cancer. George and Sykes (1997: 246–7) identify a number of ways in which terminally ill elderly people are different from younger patients. It is not simply that they are more likely to be dying from non-malignant conditions but also that they are likely 'to have multiple clinical diagnoses involving multisystem pathology'. The diagnosis that they are dying is 'often made only by exclusion, that is, after failure of standard treatment'; thus this diagnosis occurs nearer to the event of death, leaving less time for palliative care to be instigated. Communication with residents is more difficult due to confusion, dementia, impaired hearing, and vision. Residents have often lived with these chronic conditions for many years.

The unpredictable physical health and psychological and social needs of older people residing in care homes make the provision of palliative care more difficult as standard packages or pathways for care cannot be assumed. The emphasis on meeting individual need in the NSF for Older People and the National Minimum Standards makes it more complicated when planning the provision of care, because an individual's need has to be balanced with organizational logistics.

Cultures of care

The cultures of care homes are shaped by and mirror attitudes towards older people and their placement within society (Hockey 1990; Hockey and James 1993; Peace et al. 1997). Chapter 2 has considered societal ageism as well as other factors such as architecture and the design of buildings, staff morale, poor resourcing, the institutionalization of care, and attitudes towards death. The culture of a care home creates the environment within which the care for dying and living residents occurs. The extent to which this culture can influence the experience of care has long been recognized (Miller and Gwynne 1972; Bland 1999). Within nursing homes two key functions are held together in tension in a way that is not seen in residential care homes: they are both a home for the residents who live there and a place of nursing care (Froggatt 2001). OU Study (1) found that most nursing homes deliberately referred to their residents as patients to highlight their primary focus. In contrast, residents in residential care homes who require nursing care, receive technical nursing care, for example, dressings from external nursing staff, more akin to the care offered to people living in their own homes. The care home is therefore primarily a home, rather than a place where sick people can be looked after.

The management of death and dying within care homes exemplifies the underlying cultural context further. Where death is accepted and integrated with living, as may be seen particularly in homes run by religious organizations (Sidell *et al.* 1997), staff, residents, and relatives may be able to talk openly about forthcoming events, including the possibility of dying. Where residents who are dying are separated from other, 'non-dying', residents the context becomes one that does not easily facilitate discussions about dying (Hockey 1990). Even where religious beliefs underpin the culture of homes as in Kellaher's study of Methodist homes the boundaries between life and death may be marshalled by residents themselves. The increasing frailty and disturbance by some residents created dilemmas for other residents who preferred it if frail residents were cared for elsewhere, whilst recognizing they would not wish to be moved were they themselves deemed to be frail (Kellaher 2000).

A particular cultural approach to an organization arises as a consequence of a number of factors, structural and resource led, but also value based. In singly owned homes the dominant role of the owner–manager or Matron can significantly shape the culture of the home. In business or religious chains of homes the prevailing cultural ethos may come from a general cultural stance to the purpose of the home and towards the care for dying residents. Many care homes are based in the independent sector and are run as businesses, with an imperative to make a profit either for the owners or the shareholders. The extent to which this basis for existence influences the ways care homes are run has not been fully explored. Comparisons might be made with voluntary hospices: although non-NHS hospices sit firmly in the independent not-for-profit sector they manage to maintain an open and accepting attitude towards death and dying.

Material factors such as architectural design, adaptations to buildings and staffing levels affect care home cultures. Many care homes occupy converted buildings which, whilst retaining home like features, do not always match new standards for the provision of space and facilities. Resource constraints such as difficulties in recruitment and retention of staff and funding problems impact upon the ability of homes and their staff to address issues of developing practice in its widest sense. The nursing and residential care home sector is likely to face continuing financial constraints and the profile of care homes is such that their closure is barely noted. The introduction of higher standards and tighter regulation, particularly the implementation of National Minimum Standards (DoH 2001a) will also have implications for the organization and cultures of care homes.

Staff skills

There are a variety of staff that provide care for residents in care homes (Fig. 11.1). In both nursing and residential homes most of the contact with and care for residents, including those who are dying, will be provided as part of their general work by low paid, mainly female, staff with little or no training or preparation for such care work (see Chapter 8). Only in nursing homes will there be trained nursing staff and health care assistants. The low level of trained staff

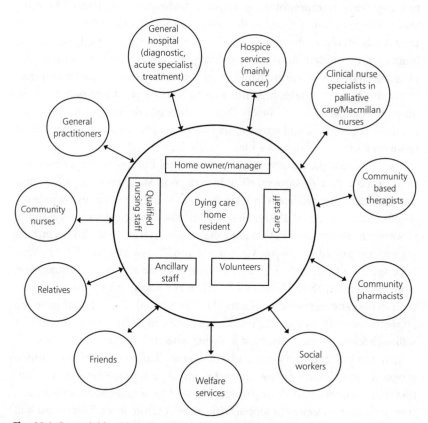

Fig. 11.1 Potential health and social care services for dying care home residents.

means that it may be difficult to manage the needs of residents living with ongoing chronic conditions and adds to the difficulties caused by the disease profile of residents for recognizing the needs of residents for palliative care. It also means that staff are unlikely to be able to meet identified palliative care needs (e.g. pain control, psychological support) and/or lack confidence to do so.

Being able to assess residents for their palliative care needs assumes that staff have an understanding of a palliative care approach and the role of and access to specialist palliative care services (see Chapter 1). OU Study (1) found such understanding was uncommon and that the understandings of palliative care held by home care staff were often related to the common perception that palliative care is concerned with (younger) cancer patients only (Sidell *et al.* 1997; Katz *et al.* 1999). Staff skills in assessment for palliative care may be limited and the assessment of older people can also be problematic because of the physical and mental conditions of the residents being assessed. Many residents in nursing and residential care homes are frail and live with multiple chronic conditions. Concurrent dementia and confusion may make it harder for staff to recognize or interpret other symptoms (Addington-Hall 2000). There are also communication difficulties that affect the ability of residents to express their needs. Staff may therefore have to rely on their own knowledge of what is 'normal' for a resident or use the knowledge of family members as indicators of change. Where residents remain in care homes for years or months this may be relatively easy to establish. Admissions to Nursing Homes of patients from hospitals that occur shortly before they die increases the difficulties of assessing in an appropriate and sensitive way how to ensure that the needs of such residents and their relatives are met.

It appears that the quality of symptom control in these settings continues to be variable, ranging from excellent to very poor. Many nursing staff are neither confident nor proficient in their ability to manage pain in dying patients (Gibbs 1995; Sidell *et al.* 1997). They may also be concerned with their ability to work effectively with health care professionals external to the home, including general practitioners (see Chapters 4 and 7). Issues of confidence have been specifically identified for care assistants in the area of communication work, particularly the ability to discuss issues of death, dying or bereavement with dying, and bereaved residents (Froggatt 2000). Even if staff have the appropriate skills to care for residents at the end of life these may not be utilized because of the problem of knowing when to use them.

As noted in Chapter 8 attendance of care staff at education and training programmes to improve their knowledge and skills is problematic, as the limited staff numbers, particularly of nursing staff in nursing homes, mean that there is little or no leeway to support paid absences from work. This means staff are often funding themselves and using their own time for their professional development. Many care staff are amongst the lowest paid workers nationally, and may be unable to meet the costs of further training (Dalley and Denniss 2000) (see Chapters 2 and 8). Staffing levels may mean that adopting a palliative care approach by, for example, ensuring there is time within the home to allow staff to spend time talking with dying residents about their concerns, and to provide support for staff during such sensitive situations may be difficult.

The understanding by home staff of a palliative approach and how to implement it in the care of dying residents is crucial to the good care of residents. Equally important is knowledge of and access to specialist palliative care services. At present general practitioners provide the main source of referral of care home residents to such services and are very influential in the care that dying residents receive (see Chapters 7 and 9). Shared informed understandings between home staff and general practitioners about palliative care and its relevance to care residents is thus another essential element for the delivery of good palliative care in care homes.

Relationships between homes, care providers, and specialist palliative care services

A crucial difficulty for the delivery of good palliative care in care homes is the complexity of working with the range of health and social welfare staff that may become involved when a resident is chronically ill with advanced disease (Fig. 11.1). This complex set of relationships has been discussed in Chapter 9. In this section we consider the main external contributors to the delivery of palliative care to residents of care homes.

Unlike hospices or other specialist palliative care units, the multidisciplinary 'team' that cares for the dying person in a care home, in so far as one exists, is largely external to the institution. Drawing upon the experience and skills of individuals from different specialisms has the potential to provide more comprehensive and effective palliative care for care home residents. However, as Ingham and Coyle (1997: 260–2) note in their discussion of the interdisciplinary team for end-of-life care, a multidisciplinary group of professionals working together does not constitute a team. They suggest the establishment of team working requires common purpose and unified identity, shared information among team members, patients and family, and understanding within the team of the responsibility and decision making capacity of each individual. They note that 'In an effective and efficient interdisciplinary team each member will have an understanding of the skills, capabilities, and roles of other members. Team leadership and responsibility are vested in the person whose expertise is most appropriate to the particular clinical situation...' (p. 161). The complexity of service relationships in the community, especially those between 'health' and 'social' services, is a potential barrier to achieving such effective team work. Field and Addington-Hall (1999) see the establishment of good working relationships between generalist and specialist providers of palliative care as an essential prerequisite of providing 'palliative care for all' (p. 1278). However, they do not discuss these points with particular reference to care homes.

There is an increasingly one-sided relationship with general hospitals, especially for nursing homes. General hospitals provide acute specialist intervention for many residents, but changes in the NHS since the 1990s have meant that nursing homes have largely replaced long stay wards for longer term symptom management and nursing care (see Chapter 2, Table 2.2). In 1999 Avis et al. reported that greater numbers of dying people were admitted to nursing homes from the NHS than previously, and in-patient hospices have also begun to refer patients for admission to nursing homes (Maccabee 1994; Williams 2000). Yet while hospitals and some hospices transfer patients with chronic/advanced diseases to nursing homes it is still the case that admission from care homes to hospitals is less likely to occur than from domestic homes. When it does occur the timing may be so close to death that it is inappropriate (Cartwright 1991; Sidell et al. 1997). More effective and reciprocal working relationships between care homes and other institutions caring for people with advanced disease conditions are essential if effective palliative care is to be provided for care home residents. In particular, greater involvement by gerontologists in such care.

George and Sykes (1997: 244) suggest that specialist palliative care services should be used in a consultative manner, usually having 'short term contacts with defined end points', with a role for palliative physicians to manage symptoms 'earlier in the disease' as part of 'full multi-disciplinary palliative care', and in terminal care in the last few days. Local hospices are potential sources for the management of difficult symptoms and for terminal care, but access to them may be difficult for care home residents, particularly those with conditions other than cancer.[1]

Few care homes in OU Study (1) used hospice and specialist palliative care services (Sidell et al. 1997; Katz et al. 1999). However, there is some evidence of involvement in nursing and residential care homes by specialist

---

[1]   The National Council for Hospice and Specialist Palliative Care Minimum data sets project 2001 covering the year April 2000–March 2001 found that of the 27, 173 in-patient hospice admissions for which there was information about their pre-admission location 177 (0.65 per cent) were from nursing or residential homes. Calculated by Ann Eve, Hospice Information Service, for this chapter.

palliative care providers, particularly Clinical Nurse Specialists (CNSs) (Froggatt *et al.* 2001). Respondents in a UK wide survey of 730 community CNSs in palliative care (Froggatt *et al.* 2001) indicated that the vast majority of them had contact with nursing homes (92 per cent of respondents) and residential care homes (80 per cent of respondents). The interaction with care home staff was usually reactive and took the form of visits to see residents or telephone support for care home staff. Residents with cancer received the most attention from CNSs, unless there was an identifiable symptom problem for a resident with another condition. The direct clinical care activities focused upon pain and symptom control, although there was evidence that some CNSs addressed psychosocial care issues as well. A few designated Clinical Nurse Specialist posts in palliative care exist in the United Kingdom that have a specific remit to work with care homes and as well as addressing resident needs reactively can also work proactively to develop palliative care practices through the development of educational courses tailored to the homes worked with. However, there is no systematic evaluation of the effectiveness of these roles to date.

As discussed in Chapter 7, general practitioners and community nurses play a vital role in the care of residents in nursing and residential homes. For example, general practitioners are the primary resource for pain control and, as noted, referral to palliative care services. Thus, it is important that general practitioners and community nurses are aware of and skilled in generic palliative care. It is recognized that it is particularly difficult for health professionals to identify patients with long-term chronic non-malignant conditions as in need of palliative care (Field 1998; Field and Addington-Hall 1999). This difficulty is likely to be more pronounced for general practitioners and district nurses visiting care homes, especially when they are infrequent visitors. Froggatt (2000) found that where care home staff are trained for palliative care, but General Practitioners are not, conflicts can occur over, for example, pain management. Community based therapists could also contribute to the palliative care of residents, although there is no clear evidence about the extent to which this occurs.

Social welfare services and care managers are potentially involved with residents at two points in their residence. They have an involvement with the assessment and placement of residents into care homes and maintain a watching brief for six weeks after. In addition established residents who have self-funded their entry into a care home may require social services support when their capital falls below the level at which state support can be sought. The assessment of their income and capital entails social services staff involvement. Community pharmacists are another group of staff who play an important, yet often under-recognized role in ensuring the good care of dying residents through their supply of appropriate controlled medication and advice to care staff.

To summarize this section, the delivery of good palliative care to residents of care homes will require cooperation between care home staff and a range of generalist and specialist care providers. This range of carers should work together to identify goals of care and how to use the skills and abilities of care providers to achieve these. This requires the understanding of the contributions each can make, effective communications and mutual respect and trust between those involved. The coordination of care is critical, especially as the patient's condition deteriorates, but is hard to achieve where 'team' members do not consistently work with each other and where there is no clear responsibility or authority for such coordination of care.

Resident experiences

One of the aims of palliative care is to enable people to participate in the choices and decisions that are made about their care. The ideal is that patients die a 'good death', defined in their terms rather than those of their carers. How might this central feature of palliative care be achieved in care homes? Indeed, is it possible for residents to participate in such decision making?

One area of expressed choice is the place of dying. It is now well established that in the United Kingdom people would prefer to die at home rather than in a hospital (Townsend *et al.* 1990; Hinton 1994). However, this has not been established for residents living in care homes although, as Lloyd (2000) found, this may well be the case. Entry to a nursing home and, especially, into a residential home is often seen by the new elderly resident as the final move of their life, but it is frequently unclear how residents want or expect to be cared for when they come to die. Some homes try to gain such information from residents upon admission to the home, but this is often felt to be difficult by home staff. For example, Froggatt (2000) noted that staff would frequently wait until residents were settled in the home before attempting to address sensitive issues around their preferences for care at the end and after life. In any case, the views of residents may change over time, especially during the period of their general deterioration and subsequent dying when this takes place over a long time.

Another important area of decision making concerns the management of physical symptoms. A significant minority of residents may be confused or unable to communicate, thus making it difficult for home staff to establish what their wishes are, emphasizing the need to ascertain preferences for such residents before dementia becomes severe (see Chapter 5; Lloyd 2000).

However, many residents are mentally alert and fully able to participate in such decisions, providing staff are both able to recognize that the resident is dying or likely to die in the foreseeable future and willing *and* able to discuss the resident's wishes with them. Unfortunately, as noted earlier in this book, many staff, especially untrained care staff, are not sufficiently skilled in either of these areas. Even when staff are willing to discuss wishes with residents it may be difficult to do so in care homes where the culture emphasizes 'living' and ignores or denies 'dying'.

Directions for the future

A number of issues have been identified that impact upon the delivery of generic palliative care to residents in care homes. In asking staff to address the palliative care needs of their residents it must be recognized that the dying resident will only be one of many other residents whose needs concern living within the care home. To incorporate the care of dying residents within this wider milieu may therefore require paradigmatic shifts in understandings about the purpose of care in such institutions. This diverse population means that the delivery of good palliative care is harder than in hospices, where the client group is much more homogeneous and efforts can be focused upon living while dying.

Education

In the United Kingdom the main attempts to improve palliative care for care home residents have been through the education of home staff. However, the efficacy of such initiatives has yet to be clearly demonstrated. What is clear is that education alone is insufficient (Froggatt 2001a). As a result of her evaluative study of providing education for palliative care to nursing home staff, Froggatt (2000, 2001a) found that both nursing staff and aide workers benefited from their courses, but that implementing their learning into practice depended upon the culture of the home and whether they were supported by their managers in their palliative care work. She concluded that education is a necessary, but insufficient route to improving palliative care within nursing homes. Both the Open University studies and the research by Froggatt make it clear that education needs to be targeted more broadly than at trained nursing staff, especially in residential care homes. It is also clear that the financial and time costs of such education to homes and staff may be a disincentive to participation and that for maximal effect education should be provided either within or very close to the care home.

Unlike hospices, who developed and provided education and training on the basis of their practice knowledge, UK care homes have been primarily recipients rather than providers of education about palliative care. This is changing as placements of nursing students are occurring within nursing homes as a result of the closure of long stay care settings for older people within the NHS. There have also been calls for the creation of 'teaching' nursing homes where multi disciplinary learning by medical, nursing, social work, and allied health professionals could occur (Joint Working Party 2000). Good palliative care draws upon more general skills and attitudes towards patient care. Thus the further development of such general education could prove beneficial to the delivery of palliative care as general standards of care improve through the involvement of care homes in the training, mentoring and quality assurance systems of departments of nursing, and their Higher Education Institutions. However, the lack of qualified nursing staff in residential homes means that these are further distanced from such educational initiatives.

Collaborative models for palliative care in care homes

In the modern hospice movement practice has been enhanced by research to create knowledge that underpins the care offered. Applying this model to care homes, we can see that there are no well-recognized 'demonstration models' for good practice, that research has only recently begun, and that it is mainly restricted to nursing homes. Here we briefly summarize collaborative models for delivering palliative care for care home residents from the United Kingdom, Australia, and Canada.

In the United Kingdom the Joint Working Party (2000) on the health and care of older people in care homes has recommended the need for the development of Gerontological Nurse Specialists (GNS) to be the lead clinical practitioner for health care support in care homes. There have also been calls for the creation of clinical nurse specialists (CNS) in palliative care to work specifically with care homes (Froggatt 2001a). It has been proposed that these CNSs would have responsibility for developing and supporting practice in palliative care within a number of nursing and residential care homes. In May 2002 comparatively few posts like these existed within the United Kingdom and formal evaluative work of the efficacy of their role has yet to be undertaken. The success of such proposed posts would depend upon successful working with general practitioners and care home staff. The role of specialist palliative care practitioners in care homes needs to be considered carefully, especially how palliative care principles and practices apply in these contexts which have a very different population of dying people and a different approach to dying people. The establishment of partnerships between the CNS and the GNS to create a dynamic resource for the care homes in end-of-life care would be a model worth evaluating.

We noted earlier that in the UK hospices have begun to refer patients for admission to nursing homes, a practice that seems likely to become more common as in-patient hospices increasingly come to be used primarily for short-term crisis intervention and terminal care in the last few days of life. In 1994 Maccabee suggested that the establishment of nursing home annexes to hospices would ease the transition from hospice to nursing home by providing continuity of care and enhancing palliative care in nursing homes. Maddocks and Parker (2001) report on such an arrangement established in Adelaide, Australia, in 1997. Here a nursing home has agreed with an adjacent in-patient hospice to give priority to clients from the palliative care programme who qualify for admission to the nursing home. Following transfer the palliative care team maintain regular contact with the resident and their family. Nursing home staff receive training in palliative care and a general practitioner with experience in palliative care also provides care. As of April 2002 this arrangement was still in place, with weekly visits to the nursing home by a palliative care physician as required, three monthly meetings between the director of nursing and community clinical nurse consultants, and access to social work support. However, nursing home beds are not always available for hospice patients who thus have to be transferred elsewhere.[2] Unfortunately no formal evaluation of the arrangement has been conducted, as this model seems well worth considering (as Maccabee suggested) in the United Kingdom.

In Canada work is devolved to the Provinces and consequently varies across the country. Although all facilities that offer long-term care will offer end-of-life care they are not all equipped to provide palliative care. A National Guide for End-of-Life Care for Seniors (Ross *et al.* 2000) has been produced that offers guidance of relevance to long-term care facilities within Canada. The guide provides an account of best practice in the care of older people with progressive or chronic life threatening conditions at the end of their lives. Although not focused directly upon care homes, it aims to increase the capacity of the community to provide end-of-life care of a high standard for older people and their families across a range of settings, including care homes. The guide is the product of an active collaboration between palliative care, gerontology and user groups representing older people. It is being used in some Provinces to drive initiatives forward, for example, in Winnipeg.

Research

Research into care homes is almost always initiated by people external to them, rather than initiated by them (but see Froggatt (2000)), which means

---

[2]   Information provided by D. Parker, Department of Palliative and Supportive Care, School of Medicine, Flinders University of South Australia.

that the expertise and requirements of care homes are not always adequately represented in the development of research. What is needed is to set up a range of different models for palliative care, and to subject these to research scrutiny. This would require the cooperation of a range of interested parties, including care homes, and substantial funding.

Different models of palliative care for residents should be researched, and methods of symptom management developed that recognize the dependence of effective palliative care in these settings upon its continuity with care provided to residents living with long-term conditions. Education in palliative care for care staff must reflect the pattern of dying in care homes and be based upon the experiences of care staff drawing upon their experiences and skills. There are a number of ongoing initiatives within palliative care and gerontology to address the issue of high quality care for care residents but at the time of writing (May 2002) no results have been published.

Conclusion

The nature of care practices within care homes is largely determined by the particular location of these institutions within the health and social care systems of the United Kingdom. Care homes are positioned on the boundaries of a number of domains. The vast majority of them are situated in the private and not-for-profit sectors, rather than in the public sector as seen in Chapter 2. They also straddle the boundary between health and social care. Unlike hospice care, which has a high public regard, the care offered in care homes is often perceived to be of a poor standard (Royal College of Nursing 1992; Centre for Policy on Ageing 1996; Peace *et al*. 1997). In some instances the deficits in care are justifiably raised, and can be partly attributed to endemic low levels of funding that create a context of resource constraints. Another contributory factor can be the 'cultures of care' within some care homes that emphasize life and living but do not fully integrate care work associated with dying into home life. The combination of financial constraints and the emphasis on life shapes the way in which good palliative care can be provided for residents.

It is our argument that palliative care within care homes must be generic in nature and that it can only be delivered effectively by 'generalists' who are supported in their care by specialists. The emphasis should be upon ensuring and improving the delivery of generic palliative care within homes provided through home-based nursing staff and district nursing and general practitioner services, supported by specialist palliative care services in the community. Collaborative initiatives between specialist palliative nursing, gerontology, and care homes seem to offer a route to care that integrates the needs of both living and dying residents. It may well be that it is in such partnerships that the future lies.

References

Addington-Hall, J. (2000) *Positive Partnerships Palliative Care for Adults with Severe Mental Health Problems*. National Council for Hospice and Specialist Palliative Care Services and Scottish partnership Agency for Palliative and Cancer Care, London.

Avis, M., Jackson, J.G., Cox, C., and Miskella, C. (1999) Evaluation of a project providing community palliative care support to nursing homes. *Health and Social Care in the Community*, 7, 32–8.

Bland, R. (1999) Independence, privacy and risk: Two contrasting approaches to residential care for older people. *Ageing and Society*, 18, 539–60.

Cartwright, A. (1991) The role of residential and nursing homes in the last year of people's lives. *British Journal of Social Work*, 21, 81–7.

Centre for Policy on Ageing. (1996) *A Better Home Life. A Code of Good Practice for Residential and Nursing Homes*. Centre for Policy on Ageing, London.

Clark, D. and Seymour, J. (1999) *Reflections on Palliative Care*. Open University Press, Buckingham.

Dalley, G. and Denniss, M. (2000) *Trained to Care? Investigating the Skills and Competencies of Care Assistants in Homes for Older People*. Centre for Policy on Ageing, London.

Davies, S., Slack, R., Laker, S., and Philp, I. (2000) The educational preparation of staff in nursing homes: Relationship with resident autonomy. *Journal of Advanced Nursing*, 29(1), 208–17.

Department of Health. (2000a) *The NHS Cancer Plan*. A Plan for Investment A Plan for Reform. Department of Health, London.

Department of Health. (2000b) *National Service Framework for Coronary Heart Disease*. Department of Health, London.

Department of Health. (2001a) *Care Homes for Older People* National Minimum Standards. The Stationery Office, London.

Department of Health. (2001b) *National Service Framework for Older People*. Department of Health, London.

Eve, A. and Smith, A.M. (1996) Survey of hospice and palliative care inpatient units in the UK and Ireland, 1993. *Palliative Medicine*, 10, 13–21.

Field, D. (1998) Special not different: General practitioners' accounts of their care of dying people. *Social Science and Medicine*, 46, 1111–20.

Field, D. (2000) Older people's attitudes towards death in England. *Mortality*, 5, 277–97.

Field, D. and Addington-Hall, J. (1999) Extending specialist palliative care to all? *Social Science and Medicine*, 48, 1271–80.

Field, D. and James, V. (1993) Where and how people die, in D. Clark (ed.) *The Future for Palliative Care. Issues of Policy and Practice*. Open University Press, Buckingham, 6–29.

Froggatt, K.A. (2000) *Palliative Care Education in Nursing Homes*. Macmillan Cancer Relief, London.

Froggatt, K.A. (2001a) Palliative care in nursing homes: Where next? *Palliative Medicine*, 15, 42–8.

Froggatt, K.A. (2001b) Life and death in English nursing homes: Sequestration or transition? *Ageing and Society*, 21, 319–32.

Froggatt, K.A., Poole, K., and Hoult, E. (2001) *Community Work with Nursing Homes and Residential Care Homes: A Survey Study of Clinical Nurse Specialists in Palliative Care*. Macmillan Cancer Relief, London.

George, R. and Sykes, J. (1997) Beyond cancer?, in D. Clark *et al.* (eds) *New Themes in Palliative Care*. Open University Press, Buckingham, 239–54.

Gibbs, G. (1995) Nurses in private nursing homes: a study of their knowledge and attitudes to pain management in palliative care. *Palliative Medicine*, **9**, 245–53.

Hinton, J. (1994) Can home care maintain an acceptable quality of life for patients with terminal illness and their families? *Palliative Medicine*, **8**, 183–96.

Hockey, J. (1990) *Experiences of Death*. Edinburgh University Press, Edinburgh.

Hockey, J. and James, A. (1993) *Growing Up and Growing Old: Ageing and Dependency in the Life Course*. Sage, London.

Ingham, J.M. and Coyle, N. (1997) Teamwork in end-of-life care: A nurse–physician perspective on introducing physicians to palliative care concepts, in D. Clark *et al.* (eds) *New Themes in Palliative Care*. Open University Press, Buckingham, 255–74.

Joint Working Party. (2000) *The Health and Care of Older People in Care Homes. A Comprehensive Interdisciplinary Approach*. Royal College of Physicians, Royal College of Nursing, and British Geriatrics Society, London.

Katz, J., Komaromy, C., and Sidell, M. (1999) Understanding palliative care in residential and nursing homes. *International Journal of Palliative Nursing*, **5**, 58–64.

Kellaher, L. (2000) *A Choice Well Made. 'Mutuality' as a Governing Principle in Residential Care*. Centre for Policy on Aging/Methodist Homes, London.

Lloyd, L. (2000) Dying in old age: Promoting well-being at the end of life. *Mortality*, **5**, 171–88.

Maccabee, J. (1994) The effect of transfer from a palliative care unit to nursing homes—are patients' and relatives' needs met? *Palliative Medicine*, **8**, 211–14.

Maddocks, I. and Parker, D. (2001) Palliative care in nursing homes, in J. Addington-Hall and I. Higginson (eds) *Palliative Care for Non-Cancer Patients*. Oxford University Press, Oxford, 147–57.

Mellor, P.A. and Shilling, C. (1993). Modernity, self-identity and the sequestration of death. *Sociology*, **27**(3), 411–31.

Miller, E.J. and Gwynne, G.V. (1972) *A Life Apart. A Pilot Study of Residential Institutions for the Physically Handicapped and the Young Chronic Sick*. Tavistock, London.

Miskella, C. and Avis, M. (1998) Care of the dying person in the nursing home: Exploring the care assistants' contribution. *European Journal Oncology Nursing*, **2**, 80–6.

National Association of Health Authorities and Trusts. (1991) *Care of People with a Terminal Illness*. A Report by the Joint Advisory Group. NAHAT, Birmingham.

NCHSPCS (1995) *Specialist Palliative Care: A Statement of Definitions*. National Council for Hospice and Specialist Palliative Care Services, London.

Peace, S.M., Kellaher, L., and Willcocks, D. (1997) *Re-evaluating Residential Care*. Open University Press, Buckingham.

Ross, M.M., Fisher, R., and Maclean, M.J. (2000) End-of-life care for seniors: The development of a national guide. *Journal of Palliative Care*, **16**(4), 47–53.

Royal College of Nursing. (1992) *A Scandal Waiting to Happen*? Royal College of Nursing, London.

Shemmings, Y. (1996) *Death, Dying and Residential Care*. Avebury, Aldershot.

Sidell, M., Katz, J.T., and Komaromy, C. (1997) *Dying in Nursing and Residential Nursing Homes for Older People: Examining the Case for Palliative Care.* Report for the Department of Health. Open University, Milton Keynes.

Townsend, J., Frank, O.O., Fermont, D., *et al.* (1990) Terminal cancer care and patients' preference for place of death: A prospective study. *British Medical Journal,* 301, 415–17.

Williams, M. (2000) *The Transfer of Palliative Care Patients to Nursing Homes.* St Christopher's Hospice, London.

World Health Organisation. (1990) *Cancer Pain Relief and Palliative Care,* Technical report Series 804. World Health Organisation, Geneva.

Chapter 12

End of life in care homes

Sheila Peace and Jeanne Katz

Once someone is dead there is nothing you can do for them but you are still very conscious that you have a responsibility and a need to look after the living and that is the rule that all the staff work by.

In care homes is the denial of death the ultimate ageism? In this book the authors have each contributed to a broader understanding of the end of life for older people in care homes through the experiences of those older people themselves, care staff, family and friends, other residents, and external health care workers. Fundamental to this discussion has been an acknowledgement of the parallel experiences of residents as they reach the end of their lives within collective accommodation—living yet dying over a period of time which may be short or long. Is this the reason why has it taken so long to be recognized?

We have seen how the histories of residential care homes and nursing homes have followed different paths for different people; the one beginning with the needs of the unemployed working class poor, the other with the health care needs of a more affluent group—coming together through the emergence of a National Health Service and provision of accommodation and care. More recently a gradual awareness of the needs of an ageing society facing family and household change is transforming the reality of long-term care for some people at the end of life.

Acknowledging that some older people will always live collectively outside their private domestic home and that more may chose to do so, has led policy-makers and researchers to question the circumstances in which this takes place. Concerns have been voiced over the advantages and disadvantages of individual v collective living with attention focused on the material environment, daily routines, social relations, activity, and community participation—aspects of daily living where the older person remains engaged. The focus has been on developing a culture of care which enhances the quality of life valuing the individual and avoiding institutionalization.

Yet the characteristics of residents have also been changing: getting older; becoming more culturally diverse; maintaining chronic health conditions that have become part of life; becoming more cognitively impaired and more vulnerable. The reality for many people is chronicity and mental frailty. Whilst no one will deny that the quality of life needs to improve for these older people the uneven boundary between life and death needs to be acknowledged and the quality of death given equal recognition.

How is this to happen? This text has given us much to think about and several specific suggestions have already been made in Chapter 11. Fundamental are two factors: relationships and resources.

Relationships

Throughout this book we have seen that there are many relationships in care homes: between care staff and residents; residents and family and friends; care staff and family; between residents themselves; managerial and care staff at all levels; care home staff and external health workers, and each of these relationships may have an impact on the person who is dying and their death.

In Chapters 4 and 5 we noted how care staff can in many ways become surrogate family for some residents. Most of the time they are engaged in the business of maintaining the daily routine for people living their everyday lives and often managing chronic health conditions. In parallel some will be involved with people whose circumstances mean that they are beginning to disengage from daily life or fluctuate between engagement and disengagement. In Chapter 3, we viewed this dying trajectory, the uncertainty of the commencement of which needs greater understanding and recognition. Disengagement involves staff in watching and listening—with some more conscious of dying and death than others.

The collectivity of care is also important in understanding the development of relationships in care homes. There is a tension between the quality of individual life and group life which feeds on resources and impacts on underlying values and attitudes. The person-centred approach to care can be supported through a philosophy that is underpinned by values and fostered through training and systems such as key-working. Such developments can only be of benefit to the group of older people living alongside each other and to encouraging greater openness between residents themselves and between residents and their families, if not the local community.

Openness about dying and death does not mean that it has to become dominant rather an acknowledgement that it happens. We have seen that in many homes residents are shielded from this information and yet those who 'want to know, get to know'. It may be true that many residents are 'not afraid' of death and might welcome the opportunity to talk about it. Yet even small qualitative research studies undertaken in the United States suggest that it is not at all clear that older people do want to discuss death or plan for end-of-life care despite the increasing popularity of advance directives (Winland-Brown 1998; Carrese *et al.* 2002). This is a tension faced by informal and formal carers in all environments. Chapter 8 demonstrated that communication is a key issue within training and throughout this book we have noted that many carers find it difficult knowing how to talk about death. We have also seen how people may welcome opportunities to discuss or listen to issues of spirituality and existential feelings without necessarily being part of a denominational religious group. Yet we have recognized the different ways in which both cultural and religious factors can affect how dying and death are valued in some homes.

But whilst we have seen that positive relationships do develop within care homes we have also noted both the ability, and the lack of ability, amongst staff to improve the circumstances of an older person at the end of life, regardless of whether that person is defined as dying. Here chronicity can become invisibility; people may have suffered for a long time which may hide pain that could be treated—only it fails to be recognized without close observation. This is the point when the relationships amongst and between care home staff and other health and social care workers such as community nurses, GPs, and social workers becomes important. In Chapter 4 we saw how a majority of care home managers, let alone the carers at the front line, failed to understand the concept of palliative care. In Chapter 9 we considered positive, and not so positive, relationships with a number of GPs and saw how commitment and spending time with care staff were important to developing teamwork relationships. In this way the contribution and skills of care home staff can be acknowledged by GPs and vice versa.

In discussing these issues we also begin to recognize the relationships that exist between parts of bigger institutions—care homes and health services including specialist palliative care services. As we have seen in Chapters 1 and 11 we are gradually understanding the value of and development of palliative care for people at the end of a long life where their health needs may be multiple. We also need health staff to have greater recognition of care homes and other assisted living settings as places where some older people will live and end their lives. They need to be seen as legitimate places to be rather than places which can still project an image of 'social death' at the front door.

These are just some of the relationships which underpin the end of life in care homes and as we saw in Chapters 2 and 11, the values on which many of them are based are beginning to find their way into official guidance: National Service Frameworks, National Minimum Standards, and Codes of Practice. Whilst we would not argue that all of these policy developments will only occur through an increase in resources, we are conscious of the impact that resources can have and so it is to this area that we now turn.

Resources

In Chapter 2 we saw that over time there have been enormous changes in both the growth of residential care homes and nursing homes and their ownership, with the present dominance of the independent sector—particularly private for-profit facilities (see Table 2.2 in Chapter 2). The nature of long-term care facilities are also diverse ranging from large limited companies which own national chains of residential care and nursing homes through to small owners running one or a few homes (Laing 2002).

Following dramatic growth, the number of homes has declined more recently. This has been due partly to the implementation of the NHS and Community Care Act 1990, enormous pressure due to reduced public subsidies, and rising costs influenced by the call to meet National Minimum Standards. Proprietors of a small number of homes have become particularly vulnerable and there have been home closures. This decline in homes sits alongside policy development which seeks to enable older people to remain in their own homes for longer through rehabilitative services and direct payments for services at home (Carvel 2002).

Changes in the overall number of homes could be viewed in two ways, *either* that decline may lead to specialization, a small number of large corporations, and greater investment made on staffing, environment, and other key resources *or* that the situation continues as at present with a wide variety of forms of accommodation and a dominance of low paid, untrained, female care staff. Quality of care requires resources. Previous attempts at improving quality of life within homes have included developments based on changes in organizational and environmental structure but these demand adequate staffing to facilitate a particular philosophy (Peace *et al.* 1997).

Whilst providers may increase fees the demands on income are high. In order for practice issues surrounding the dying and death of residents to form part of the agenda they need to become part of the everyday: recognized and not hidden. In this way improvements in quality of life will also affect improvements in quality of dying and death.

Addington-Hall and Higginson (2001) note that older people with cancer, regardless of the setting in which they find themselves, have less access to hospice and palliative care services than younger people. In the United Kingdom three-quarters of those who die of cancer are over 65 however only 65 per cent of those accessing specialist palliative care team support are of this age (ibid.) Some of those older people dying of cancer live in residential and nursing homes and yet they constitute a small proportion of that population needing supportive or palliative care. These are strong arguments for the provision of additional supportive or palliative care services to long-term care facilities through the proposed geriatric nursing service and/or the clinical nurse specialists described in Chapter 11.

Education about palliative care is central to improving end-of-life care for people dying in these settings. As Chapter 8 demonstrated, there is a need for both public and private support for training in palliative care in long-term care and early referral should be a central plank of such training (Casarett *et al.* 2001). Training programmes should encompass not only care home staff but also external health and social care workers such as general practitioners, community nurses, and social workers who may also lack these skills. In addition there is a need for specialist palliative care staff to strive for an equal partnership with care home staff which recognizes the strengths and values of each party.

To conclude, one of the reasons that dying and death has been all too frequently ignored by those involved with residential services is that energy has been spent seeking to raise the profile of valuing older people's lives whilst almost forgetting to value them as they approach death. We have seen how these issues are now being taken on board in other countries with Chapters 10 and 11 demonstrating developments within the United States and Australia. Whilst we do not find ourselves in the position of placing a direct financial value on palliative care for nursing home residents who must leave aside the right to active life sustaining treatment, resourcing continues to play an indirect role within the United Kingdom.

What then do we strive for? In Chapter 3, Sidell and Komaromy utilized work by Travis *et al.* (2001) to demonstrate the concept of 'blended care', a holistic approach which expands the culture of end-of-life care to embrace living while dying. We would like to move beyond this position to a philosophical approach that can transcend the boundaries of living and dying. There should be no difference in the quality of care provided to residents regardless of whether they are living with chronic conditions or defined as dying. To answer the question that we posed at the beginning of this Chapter—it is *pervasive ageism* that must be overcome. It is this that we seek and we recognize the need to bring gerontologists and thanatologists together to address these issues further.

References

Addington-Hall, J.M., and Higginson, I.J. (2001) Discussion in Addington-Hall, J.M. and Higginson, I.J. (Eds) *Palliative Care for Non-Cancer Patients.* Oxford University Press, Oxford.

Carrese, J.A., Mullaney, J.L. Faden, R., and Finucane, T.E. (2002) Planning for death but not serious future illness: qualitative study of housebound elderly patients. *British Medical Journal,* **325**, 125–7.

Carvel, J. (2002) Elderly to get option to buy home care. *The Guardian*, July 24th, 2002, 9.

Casarett, D.J., Hirschman, K.B., and Henry, M.R. (2001) Does hospice have a role in nursing home care at the end of life? *Journal of the American Geriatric Society*, 49, 1493–8.

Laing, W. (2002) *Healthcare Market Survey 2001–2002*. Laing and Buisson, London.

Peace, S., Kellaher, L., and Willcocks, D. (1997) *Re-evaluating Residential Care*. Open University Press, Buckingham.

Travis, S.S., Loving, G., McClanahan, L., and Bernard, M. (2001) Hospitalization patterns and palliation in the last year of life among residents in long-term care. *The Gerontologist*, 41(2), 153–60.

Winland-Brown, J. (1998) Death; denial and defeat: Elders and advance directives. *Advanced Practice Nursing Quarterly*, 4(2), 36–40.

Index